BLACKWELL'S
UNDERGROUND CLINICAL VIGNETTES

PSYCHIATRY, 2E

BLACKWELL'S
UNDERGROUND CLINICAL VIGNETTES

PSYCHIATRY, 2E

VIKAS BHUSHAN, MD
University of California, San Francisco, Class of 1991
Series Editor, Diagnostic Radiologist

VISHAL PALL, MBBS
Government Medical College, Chandigarh, India, Class of 1996
Series Editor, U. of Texas, Galveston, Resident in Internal Medicine &
Preventive Medicine

TAO LE, MD
University of California, San Francisco, Class of 1996

VLADIMIR CORIC, MD
Yale University School of Medicine, Fellow in Psychiatry

LOUIS SANFILIPPO, MD
Yale University School of Medicine, Resident in Psychiatry

Blackwell
Science

CONTRIBUTORS

Siddarth Shah, MD
Mt. Sinai School of Medicine, New York, Resident in Preventive and Community Medicine

Ishnella Azad, MD
University of California, Los Angeles, Resident in Psychiatry

Fadi Abu Shahin, MD
University of Damascus, Syria, Class of 1999

Chris Aiken, MD
Yale University School of Medicine, Class of 1999

Sunit Das, MD
Northwestern University, Class of 2000

Hoang Nguyen, MD, MBA
Northwestern University, Class of 2001

© 2002 by Blackwell Science, Inc.

Editorial Offices:
Commerce Place, 350 Main Street, Malden,
    Massachusetts 02148, USA
Osney Mead, Oxford OX2 0EL, England
25 John Street, London WC1N 2BS, England
23 Ainslie Place, Edinburgh EH3 6AJ, Scotland
54 University Street, Carlton, Victoria 3053,
    Australia

Other Editorial Offices:
Blackwell Wissenschafts-Verlag GmbH,
    Kurfürstendamm 57, 10707 Berlin, Germany
Blackwell Science KK, MG Kodenmacho Building,
    7-10 Kodenmacho Nihombashi, Chuo-ku,
    Tokyo 104, Japan
Iowa State University Press, A Blackwell Science
    Company, 2121 S. State Avenue, Ames, Iowa
    50014-8300, USA

Distributors:
The Americas
Blackwell Publishing
c/o AIDC
P.O. Box 20
50 Winter Sport Lane
Williston, VT 05495-0020
(Telephone orders: 800-216-2522;
    fax orders: 802-864-7626)
Australia
Blackwell Science Pty, Ltd.
54 University Street
Carlton, Victoria 3053
(Telephone orders: 03-9347-0300;
    fax orders: 03-9349-3016)
Outside The Americas and Australia
Blackwell Science, Ltd.
c/o Marston Book Services, Ltd.
P.O. Box 269
Abingdon
Oxon OX14 4YN
England
(Telephone orders: 44-01235-465500;
    fax orders: 44-01235-465555)

Acquisitions: Laura DeYoung
Development: Amy Nuttbrock
Production: Lorna Hind and Shawn Girsberger
Manufacturing: Lisa Flanagan
Marketing Manager: Kathleen Mulcahy
Cover design by Leslie Haimes
Interior design by Shawn Girsberger
Typeset by TechBooks
Printed and bound by Capital City Press

Blackwell's Underground Clinical Vignettes:
    Psychiatry, 2e
ISBN 0-632-04573-6

Printed in the United States of America
02 03 04 05 5 4 3 2 1

The Blackwell Science logo is a trade mark of
Blackwell Science Ltd., registered at the United
Kingdom Trade Marks Registry

Library of Congress Cataloging-in-Publication Data
Bhushan, Vikas.
Blackwell's underground clinical vignettes.
Psychiatry / author, Vikas Bhushan. – 2nd ed.
    p. ; cm. – (Underground clinical vignettes)
Rev. ed. of: Psychiatry / Vikas Bhushan ... [et al.].
c1999. ISBN 0-632-04573-6 (pbk.)
1. Psychiatry – Case studies. 2. Physicians – Licenses –
United States – Examinations – Study guides.
    [DNLM: 1. Mental Disorders – Case Report.
2. Mental Disorders – Problems and Exercises.
WM 18.2 B575b 2002] I. Title: Underground clinical
vignettes. Psychiatry. II. Title: Psychiatry. III. Psychiatry.
IV. Title. V. Series.
    RC465 .B526 2002
    616.89'0076–dc21

                                    2001004889

CONTENTS

ACKNOWLEDGMENTS

Throughout the production of this book, we have had the support of many friends and colleagues. Special thanks to our support team including Anu Gupta, Andrea Fellows, Anastasia Anderson, Srishti Gupta, Mona Pall, Jonathan Kirsch and Chirag Amin. For prior contributions we thank Gianni Le Nguyen, Tarun Mathur, Alex Grimm, Sonia Santos and Elizabeth Sanders.

We have enjoyed working with a world-class international publishing group at Blackwell Science, including Laura DeYoung, Amy Nuttbrock, Lisa Flanagan, Shawn Girsberger, Lorna Hind and Gordon Tibbitts. For help with securing images for the entire series we also thank Lee Martin, Kristopher Jones, Tina Panizzi and Peter Anderson at the University of Alabama, the Armed Forces Institute of Pathology, and many of our fellow Blackwell Science authors.

For submitting comments, corrections, editing, proofreading, and assistance across all of the vignette titles in all editions, we collectively thank:

Tara Adamovich, Carolyn Alexander, Kris Alden, Henry E. Aryan, Lynman Bacolor, Natalie Barteneva, Dean Bartholomew, Debashish Behera, Sumit Bhatia, Sanjay Bindra, Dave Brinton, Julianne Brown, Alexander Brownie, Tamara Callahan, David Canes, Bryan Casey, Aaron Caughey, Hebert Chen, Jonathan Cheng, Arnold Cheung, Arnold Chin, Simion Chiosea, Yoon Cho, Samuel Chung, Gretchen Conant, Vladimir Coric, Christopher Cosgrove, Ronald Cowan, Karekin R. Cunningham, A. Sean Dalley, Rama Dandamudi, Sunit Das, Ryan Armando Dave, John David, Emmanuel de la Cruz, Robert DeMello, Navneet Dhillon, Sharmila Dissanaike, David Donson, Adolf Etchegaray, Alea Eusebio, Priscilla A. Frase, David Frenz, Kristin Gaumer, Yohannes Gebreegziabher, Anil Gehi, Tony George, L.M. Gotanco, Parul Goyal, Alex Grimm, Rajeev Gupta, Ahmad Halim, Sue Hall, David Hasselbacher, Tamra Heimert, Michelle Higley, Dan Hoit, Eric Jackson, Tim Jackson, Sundar Jayaraman, Pei-Ni Jone, Aarchan Joshi, Rajni K. Jutla, Faiyaz Kapadi, Seth Karp, Aaron S. Kesselheim, Sana Khan, Andrew Pin-wei Ko, Francis Kong, Paul Konitzky, Warren S. Krackov, Benjamin H.S. Lau, Ann LaCasce, Connie Lee, Scott Lee, Guillermo Lehmann, Kevin Leung, Paul Levett, Warren Levinson, Eric Ley, Ken Lin,

Pavel Lobanov, J. Mark Maddox, Aram Mardian, Samir Mehta, Gil Melmed, Joe Messina, Robert Mosca, Michael Murphy, Vivek Nandkarni, Siva Naraynan, Carvell Nguyen, Linh Nguyen, Deanna Nobleza, Craig Nodurft, George Noumi, Darin T. Okuda, Adam L. Palance, Paul Pamphrus, Jinha Park, Sonny Patel, Ricardo Pietrobon, Riva L. Rahl, Aashita Randeria, Rachan Reddy, Beatriu Reig, Marilou Reyes, Jeremy Richmon, Tai Roe, Rick Roller, Rajiv Roy, Diego Ruiz, Anthony Russell, Sanjay Sahgal, Urmimala Sarkar, John Schilling, Isabell Schmitt, Daren Schuhmacher, Sonal Shah, Edie Shen, Justin Smith, John Stulak, Lillian Su, Julie Sundaram, Rita Suri, Seth Sweetser, Antonio Talayero, Merita Tan, Mark Tanaka, Eric Taylor, Jess Thompson, Indi Trehan, Raymond Turner, Okafo Uchenna, Eric Uyguanco, Richa Varma, John Wages, Alan Wang, Eunice Wang, Andy Weiss, Amy Williams, Brian Yang, Hany Zaky, Ashraf Zaman and David Zipf.

For generously contributing images to the entire *Underground Clinical Vignette* Step 2 series, we collectively thank the staff at Blackwell Science in Oxford, Boston, and Berlin as well as:

- Alfred Cuschieri, Thomas P.J. Hennessy, Roger M. Greenhalgh, David I. Rowley, Pierce A. Grace (*Clinical Surgery*, © 1996 Blackwell Science), Figures 13.23, 13.35b, 13.51, 15.13, 15.2.

- John Axford (*Medicine*, © 1996 Blackwell Science), Figures f3.10, 2.103a, 2.110b, 3.20a, 3.20b, 3.25b, 3.38a, 5.9Bi, 5.9Bii, 6.41a, 6.41b, 6.74b, 6.74c, 7.78ai, 7.78aii, 7.78b, 8.47b, 9.9e, f3.17, f3.36, f3.37, f5.27, f5.28, f5.45a, f5.48, f5.49a, f5.50, f5.65a, f5.67, f5.68, f8.27a, 10.120b, 11.63b, 11.63c, 11.68a, 11.68b, 11.68c, 12.37a, 12.37b.

- Peter Armstrong, Martin L. Wastie (*Diagnostic Imaging, 4th Edition*, © 1998 Blackwell Science), Figures 2.100, 2.108d, 2.109, 2.11, 2.112, 2.121, 2.122, 2.13, 2.1ba, 2.1bb, 2.36, 2.53, 2.54, 2.69a, 2.71, 2.80a, 2.81b, 2.82, 2.84a, 2.84b, 2.88, 2.89a, 2.89b, 2.90b, 2.94a, 2.94b, 2.96, 2.97, 2.98a, 2.98c, 3.11, 3.19, 3.20, 3.21, 3.22, 3.28, 3.30, 3.34, 3.35b, 3.35c, 3.36, 4.7, 4.8, 4.9, 5.29, 5.33, 5.58, 5.62, 5.63, 5.64, 5.65b, 5.66a, 5.66b, 5.69, 5.71, 5.75, 5.8, 5.9, 6.17a, 6.17b, 6.25, 6.28, 6.29c, 6.30, 7.13, 7.17a, 7.45a, 7.45b, 7.46, 7.50, 7.52, 7.53a, 7.57a, 7.58, 8.7a, 8.7b, 8.7c, 8.86, 8.8a, 8.96, 8.9a, 9.17a, 9.17b, 10.13a, 10.13b, 10.14a, 10.14b, 10.14c, 10.17a, 10.17b, 11.16b, 11.17a, 11.17b, 11.19, 11.23, 11.24, 11.2b, 11.2d, 11.30a, 11.30b, 12.12, 12.15,

12.18, 12.19, 12.3, 12.4, 12.8a, 12.8b, 13.13a, 13.18, 13.18a, 13.20, 13.22a, 13.22b, 13.29, 14.14a, 14.5, 14.6a, 15.25b, 15.29b, 15.31, 15.37, 17.4.

- N.C. Hughes-Jones, S.N. Wickramasinghe (*Lecture Notes On: Haematology, 6th Edition,* © 1996 Blackwell Science), Figures 2.1b, 2.2a, 3.14, 3.8, 4.3, 5.2b, 5.5a, 5.8, 7.1, 7.2, 7.3, 7.5, 8.1, 10.5b, 10.6, 11.1, plate 29, plate 34, plate 44, plate 45, plate 48, plate 5, plate 42.

- Thomas Grumme, Wolfgang Kluge, Konrad Kretzschmar, Andreas Roesler (*Cerebral and Spinal Computed Tomography, 3rd Edition,* © 1998 Blackwell Science), Figures 16.2b, 16.3, 16.6a, 17.1a, 18-1c, 18-5, 41.3c, 41.3d, 44.3, 46.8, 47.7, 48.2, 48.6a, 53.5, 55.2a, 55.2c, 56.2b, 57.1, 61.3a, 61.3b, 63.1a, 64.3a, 65.3c, 66.3b, 67.6, 70.1a, 70.3, 81.2a, 81.4, 82.2, 82.3, 84.6.

- P.R. Patel (*Lecture Notes On: Radiology,* © 1998 Blackwell Science), Figures 2.15, 2.16, 2.25, 2.26, 2.30, 2.31, 2.33, 2.36, 3.11, 3.16, 3.19, 3.4, 3.7, 4.19, 4.20, 4.38, 4.44, 4.45, 4.46, 4.47, 4.49, 4.5, 5.14, 5.6, 6.18, 6.19, 6.20, 6.21, 6.22, 6.31a, 6.31b, 7.18, 7.19, 7.21, 7.22, 7.32, 7.34, 7.41, 7.46a, 7.46b, 7.48, 7.49, 7.9, 8.2, 8.3, 8.4, 8.5, 8.8, 8.9, 9.12, 9.2, 9.3, 9.8, 9.9, 10.11, 10.16, 10.5.

- Ramsay Vallance (*An Atlas of Diagnostic Radiology in Gastroenterology,* © 1999 Blackwell Science), Figures 1.22, 2.57, 2.27, 2.55a, 2.58, 2.59, 2.63, 2.64, 2.65, 3.11, 3.3, 3.37, 3.39, 3.4, 4.6a, 4.8, 4.9, 5.1, 5.29, 5.63, 5.64b, 5.65b, 5.66b, 5.68a, 5.68b, 6.110, 6.15, 6.17, 6.23, 6.29b, 6.30, 6.39, 6.64a, 6.64b, 6.75, 6.78, 6.80, 7.57a, 7.57c, 7.60a, 8.17, 8.48, 8.53, 8.66, 9.11a, 9.15, 9.17, 9.23, 9.24, 9.25, 9.28, 9.30, 9.32a, 9.33, 9.43, 9.45, 9.55b, 9.57, 9.63, 9.64a, 9.64b, 9.64c, 9.66, 10.28, 10.36, 10.44, 10.6.

Please let us know if your name has been missed or misspelled and we will be happy to make the update in the next edition.

We were very pleased with the overwhelmingly positive student feedback for the 1st edition of our *Underground Clinical Vignettes* series. Well over 100,000 copies of the UCV books are in print and have been used by students all over the world.

Over the last two years we have accumulated and incorporated **over a thousand "updates"** and improvements suggested by you, our readers, including:

- many additions of specific boards and wards testable content

- deletions of redundant and overlapping cases

- reordering and reorganization of all cases in both series

- a new master index by case name in each Atlas

- correction of a few factual errors

- diagnosis and treatment updates

- addition of 5–20 new cases in every book

- and the addition of clinical exam photographs within *UCV— Anatomy*

And most important of all, the second edition sets now include two brand new **COLOR ATLAS** supplements, one for each Clinical Vignette series.

- The *UCV–Basic Science Color Atlas* (*Step 1*) includes over 250 color plates, divided into gross pathology, microscopic pathology (histology), hematology, and microbiology (smears).

- The *UCV–Clinical Science Color Atlas* (*Step 2*) has over 125 color plates, including patient images, dermatology, and funduscopy.

Each atlas image is descriptively captioned and linked to its corresponding Step 1 case, Step 2 case, and/or Step 2 MiniCase.

How Atlas Links Work:

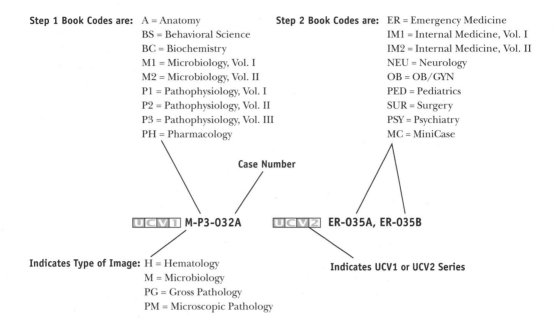

Step 1 Book Codes are:
A = Anatomy
BS = Behavioral Science
BC = Biochemistry
M1 = Microbiology, Vol. I
M2 = Microbiology, Vol. II
P1 = Pathophysiology, Vol. I
P2 = Pathophysiology, Vol. II
P3 = Pathophysiology, Vol. III
PH = Pharmacology

Step 2 Book Codes are:
ER = Emergency Medicine
IM1 = Internal Medicine, Vol. I
IM2 = Internal Medicine, Vol. II
NEU = Neurology
OB = OB/GYN
PED = Pediatrics
SUR = Surgery
PSY = Psychiatry
MC = MiniCase

Case Number

UCV1 M-P3-032A   UCV2 ER-035A, ER-035B

Indicates Type of Image:
H = Hematology
M = Microbiology
PG = Gross Pathology
PM = Microscopic Pathology

Indicates UCV1 or UCV2 Series

- If the Case number (032, 035, etc.) is not followed by a letter, then there is only one image. Otherwise A, B, C, D indicate up to 4 images.

Bold Faced Links: In order to give you access to the largest number of images possible, we have chosen to cross link the Step 1 and 2 series.

- If the link is bold-faced this indicates that the link is direct (i.e., Step 1 Case with the Basic Science Step 1 Atlas link).

- If the link is not bold-faced this indicates that the link is indirect (Step 1 case with Clinical Science Step 2 Atlas link or vice versa).

We have also implemented a few structural changes upon your request:

- Each current and future edition of our popular *First Aid for the USMLE Step 1* (Appleton & Lange/McGraw-Hill) and *First Aid for the USMLE Step 2* (Appleton & Lange/McGraw-Hill) book will be linked to the corresponding UCV case.

- We eliminated UCV → First Aid links as they frequently become out of date, as the *First Aid* books are revised yearly.

- The Color Atlas is also specially designed for quizzing—captions are descriptive and do not give away the case name directly.

New "MiniCases" replace the previous "Associated Diseases." There are now over **350 unique MiniCases** distributed throughout the *Step 2 Clinical* series, selected based on recent USMLE recollections.

We hope the updated UCV series will remain a unique and well-integrated study tool that provides compact clinical correlations to basic science information. They are designed to be easy and fun (comparatively) to read, and helpful for both licensing exams and the wards.

We invite your corrections and suggestions for the fourth edition of these books. For the first submission of each factual correction or new vignette that is selected for inclusion in the fourth edition, you will receive a personal acknowledgment in the revised book. If you submit over 20 high-quality corrections, additions or new vignettes we will also consider **inviting you to become a "Contributor" on the book of your choice**. If you are interested in becoming a potential "Contributor" or "Author" on a future UCV book, or working with our team in developing additional books, please also e-mail us your CV/resume.

We prefer that you submit corrections or suggestions via electronic mail to **UCVteam@yahoo.com**. Please include "Underground Vignettes" as the subject of your message. If you do not have access to e-mail, use the following mailing address: Blackwell Publishing, Attn: UCV Editors, 350 Main Street, Malden, MA 02148, USA.

Vikas Bhushan
Vishal Pall
Tao Le
October 2001

This series was originally developed to address the increasing number of clinical vignette questions on medical examinations, including the USMLE Step 1 and Step 2. It is also designed to supplement and complement the popular *First Aid for the USMLE Step 1* (Appleton & Lange/McGraw Hill) and *First Aid for the USMLE Step 2* (Appleton & Lange/McGraw Hill).

Each UCV 2 book uses a series of approximately 50 **"supra-prototypical" cases as a way to condense testable facts and associations**. The clinical vignettes in this series are designed to give added emphasis to pathogenesis, epidemiology, management and complications. They also contain relevant extensive B/W imaging plates within each book. Additionally, each UCV2 book contains approximately 30 to 60 "MiniCases" that focus on presenting only the key facts for that disease in a tightly edited fashion.

Although each case tends to present all the signs, symptoms, and diagnostic findings for a particular illness, **patients generally will not present with such a "complete" picture either clinically or on a medical examination**. Cases are not meant to simulate a potential real patient or an exam vignette. All the **boldfaced "buzzwords" are for learning purposes** and are not necessarily expected to be found in any one patient with the disease.

Definitions of selected important terms are placed within the vignettes in (SMALL CAPS) in parentheses. Other parenthetical remarks often refer to the pathophysiology or mechanism of disease. The format should also help students learn to present cases succinctly during oral "bullet" presentations on clinical rotations. The cases are meant to serve as a condensed review, not as a primary reference. The information provided in this book has been prepared with a great deal of thought and careful research. This book should not, however, be considered as your sole source of information. Corrections, suggestions and submissions of new cases are encouraged and will be acknowledged and incorporated when appropriate in future editions.

ABBREVIATIONS

5-ASA	5-aminosalicylic acid
ABGs	arterial blood gases
ABVD	adriamycin/bleomycin/vincristine/dacarbazine
ACE	angiotensin-converting enzyme
ACTH	adrenocorticotropic hormone
ADH	antidiuretic hormone
AFP	alpha fetal protein
AI	aortic insufficiency
AIDS	acquired immunodeficiency syndrome
ALL	acute lymphocytic leukemia
ALT	alanine transaminase
AML	acute myelogenous leukemia
ANA	antinuclear antibody
ARDS	adult respiratory distress syndrome
ASD	atrial septal defect
ASO	anti-streptolysin O
AST	aspartate transaminase
AV	arteriovenous
BE	barium enema
BP	blood pressure
BUN	blood urea nitrogen
CAD	coronary artery disease
CALLA	common acute lymphoblastic leukemia antigen
CBC	complete blood count
CHF	congestive heart failure
CK	creatine kinase
CLL	chronic lymphocytic leukemia
CML	chronic myelogenous leukemia
CMV	cytomegalovirus
CNS	central nervous system
COPD	chronic obstructive pulmonary disease
CPK	creatine phosphokinase
CSF	cerebrospinal fluid
CT	computed tomography
CVA	cerebrovascular accident
CXR	chest x-ray
DIC	disseminated intravascular coagulation
DIP	distal interphalangeal
DKA	diabetic ketoacidosis
DM	diabetes mellitus
DTRs	deep tendon reflexes
DVT	deep venous thrombosis

EBV	Epstein–Barr virus
ECG	electrocardiography
Echo	echocardiography
EF	ejection fraction
EGD	esophagogastroduodenoscopy
EMG	electromyography
ERCP	endoscopic retrograde cholangiopancreatography
ESR	erythrocyte sedimentation rate
FEV	forced expiratory volume
FNA	fine needle aspiration
FTA-ABS	fluorescent treponemal antibody absorption
FVC	forced vital capacity
GFR	glomerular filtration rate
GH	growth hormone
GI	gastrointestinal
GM-CSF	granulocyte macrophage colony stimulating factor
GU	genitourinary
HAV	hepatitis A virus
hcG	human chorionic gonadotrophin
HEENT	head, eyes, ears, nose, and throat
HIV	human immunodeficiency virus
HLA	human leukocyte antigen
HPI	history of present illness
HR	heart rate
HRIG	human rabies immune globulin
HS	hereditary spherocytosis
ID/CC	identification and chief complaint
IDDM	insulin-dependent diabetes mellitus
Ig	immunoglobulin
IGF	insulin-like growth factor
IM	intramuscular
JVP	jugular venous pressure
KUB	kidneys/ureter/bladder
LDH	lactate dehydrogenase
LES	lower esophageal sphincter
LFTs	liver function tests
LP	lumbar puncture
LV	left ventricular
LVH	left ventricular hypertrophy
Lytes	electrolytes
MCHC	mean corpuscular hemoglobin concentration
MCV	mean corpuscular volume
MEN	multiple endocrine neoplasia

MGUS	monoclonal gammopathy of undetermined significance
MHC	major histocompatibility complex
MI	myocardial infarction
MOPP	mechlorethamine/vincristine (Oncovorin)/ procarbazine/prednisone
MR	magnetic resonance (imaging)
NHL	non-Hodgkin's lymphoma
NIDDM	non-insulin-dependent diabetes mellitus
NPO	nil per os (nothing by mouth)
NSAID	nonsteroidal anti-inflammatory drug
PA	posteroanterior
PIP	proximal interphalangeal
PBS	peripheral blood smear
PE	physical exam
PFTs	pulmonary function tests
PMI	point of maximal intensity
PMN	polymorphonuclear leukocyte
PT	prothrombin time
PTCA	percutaneous transluminal angioplasty
PTH	parathyroid hormone
PTT	partial thromboplastin time
PUD	peptic ulcer disease
RBC	red blood cell
RPR	rapid plasma reagin
RR	respiratory rate
RS	Reed–Sternberg (cell)
RV	right ventricular
RVH	right ventricular hypertrophy
SBFT	small bowel follow-through
SIADH	syndrome of inappropriate secretion of ADH
SLE	systemic lupus erythematosus
STD	sexually transmitted disease
TFTs	thyroid function tests
tPA	tissue plasminogen activator
TSH	thyroid-stimulating hormone
TIBC	total iron-binding capacity
TIPS	transjugular intrahepatic portosystemic shunt
TPO	thyroid peroxidase
TSH	thyroid-stimulating hormone
TTP	thrombotic thrombocytopenic purpura
UA	urinalysis
UGI	upper GI
US	ultrasound

VDRL	Venereal Disease Research Laboratory
VS	vital signs
VT	ventricular tachycardia
WBC	white blood cell
WPW	Wolff–Parkinson–White (syndrome)
XR	x-ray

ID/CC A **73-year-old** woman who has been doing well in the hospital following an uncomplicated coronary artery bypass graft began shouting at the nurses last evening despite having been fully alert and cooperative earlier that afternoon.

HPI She pulled off her telemetry leads this morning and tried to get onto the elevator, stating, "I'm not paying for another night in this hotel; the service stinks." When redirected back to her room, she became **agitated** and assaulted a nurse. Nursing staff note that the patient has become **increasingly confused over the past several hours**. She is **arousable and responsive** but has **difficulty attending to simple commands**. She knows her name but is unsure of the year and is **unable to identify the date and season**. The patient reports that her **sleep has been erratic**, and she is not sure whether it is day or night.

PE VS: fever (39.6°C); tachycardia (HR 105); normal BP; normal RR. PE: appropriate incisional tenderness.

Labs CBC: leukocytosis (13,000). Lytes: normal. BUN, creatinine, B_{12}, folate, and TFTs normal; RPR/VDRL nonreactive. UA: moderate bacteria and leukocyte-esterase positive; urine toxicology negative. Blood cultures pending.

Pathogenesis Delirium may be secondary to a number of medical, metabolic, and drug-related factors. Anticholinergics (e.g., tricyclic antidepressants, antipsychotics, some antiparkinsonian drugs), narcotics, NSAIDs, anxiolytics, lithium, antiepileptics, beta-blockers, steroids, and digoxin are examples of some common agents that may result in **substance-induced delirium. Delirium due to a general medical condition** may result from virtually any serious medical condition, such as cardiac, neoplastic, and infectious illnesses. Neurologic diseases that may present with delirium include stroke, severe hypertension, tumor, and CNS infection. Endocrinologic causes of delirium include thyroid, adrenal, or glucose dysregulation. Common postoperative complications that may lead to delirium include fluid/electrolyte abnormalities, infections, hypoxia, sleep deprivation, pain, and stress.

Epidemiology Delirium is a common disorder, particularly on surgical services but also on general medical wards. Of hospitalized individuals older than 65 years, 10% to 15% will develop delirium during the course of their hospital stay.

DELIRIUM

Management	A **thorough medical evaluation** to identify and treat the underlying cause of delirium is critical. **Low doses** of typical **neuroleptics** (e.g., haloperidol, perphenazine) are used to manage delirium, psychosis, and agitation.
Complications	Delirium results in significant morbidity and mortality in hospitalized patients.
Differential Diagnosis	■ **Dementia** lacks the characteristic disturbance of attention that is indicative of delirium. In dementia, patients may demonstrate deficits in memory and cognition but are typically alert. The course of dementia is one of progressive decline, whereas delirium is associated with more of an acute onset with a "waxing and waning" clinical picture.
	■ **Psychotic Disorder** involves psychotic symptoms that are constant compared with delirium, in which psychosis fluctuates with the level of consciousness.
	■ **Substance Withdrawal Delirium** is diagnosed when there are derangements of attention and concentration in the setting of cessation of alcohol or sedative hypnotic use.

ID/CC A **68-year-old** retired math teacher is referred for psychiatric evaluation by her primary care physician for **progressive forgetfulness**.

HPI Her daughter notes that she has not been paying her bills on time and adds that her ability to plan ahead has been more **disorganized** (DISTURBANCE OF EXECUTIVE FUNCTIONING). She is unable to find things around the house and is more forgetful (DISTURBANCE IN MEMORY). The daughter is also worried that her mother "eats only tea and toast" and is no longer interested in activities she once enjoyed (ANHEDONIA).

PE **Alert and oriented to person, place, and year**; unable to recall specific day and month; long-term memory is intact but **short-term memory is impaired**, as evidenced by inability to recall three objects after five 5 minutes; patient has difficulty identifying objects (AGNOSIA) and performing calculations; unable to perform three-stage command or mimic complex hand gestures (APRAXIA); at times, patient demonstrates difficulty generating normal speech (APHASIA); CN II through XII intact with normal motor and sensory function throughout.

Labs Lytes/CBC: normal. TFTs normal; RPR/VDRL nonreactive. UA: toxicology negative.

Imaging CT, head (noncontrast): **diffuse cerebral atrophy** without evidence of mass, infarct, or bleed.

Pathogenesis Dementia is caused by a variety of illnesses; Alzheimer's dementia is the most common type and is associated pathologically with **neurofibrillary tangles, amyloid plaques**, and **degeneration of the nucleus basalis of Meynert**. Physiologically it is associated with **decreased central cholinergic transmission**.

Epidemiology Dementia affects approximately 15% to 20% of those over 65; in patients older than 80, severe dementia occurs with a prevalence of 25%.

Management Thorough medical evaluation is critical to **rule out treatable causes of dementia** (e.g., folate deficiency, vitamin B_{12} or B_1 deficiency, syphilis, thyroid dysfunction, vasculitis, and normal pressure hydrocephalus). Treatment for Alzheimer's dementia is largely supportive, with the aim of keeping the patient safe, educating the family, and increasing support and structure systems as clinically warranted. **Donepezil** (Aricept) and **tacrine**

DEMENTIA—ALZHEIMER'S

(Cognex) are reversible acetylcholinesterase inhibitors used in the treatment of Alzheimer's dementia (note that tacrine has been associated with hepatic failure and is less commonly used). Vascular dementia can be treated or prevented with **aspirin, estrogen replacement**, and reduction of cardiovascular risk factors. Low doses of high-potency **neuroleptics** (e.g., haloperidol) are useful in the management of the agitated dementia patient; higher doses or atypical neuroleptics should be used when psychotic symptoms are prominent. Anticholinergic agents (e.g., benztropine) and benzodiazepines should be administered cautiously because they may cause further impairment of cognition.

Complications Many patients with significant dementia develop delusions (especially the paranoid type) and hallucinations. Depression occurs in half of patients. In most dementias, deterioration occurs over 5 to 10 years, leading to death.

Atlas Links UCV1 PG-BS-005, PM-BS-005A, PM-BS-005B

Differential Diagnosis ■ **Delirium** is characterized by a gross impairment in consciousness, attention, and orientation. Furthermore, the onset of delirium is acute, and its course often fluctuates dramatically over hours or days.

■ **Multi-infarct Dementia** is the second leading cause of progressive cognitive decline and results from repeated CNS infarctions of various sizes. The clinical course of vascular dementia is often characterized by a "stepwise" decline that is thought to correlate with each successive ischemic event.

■ **Alcoholic Dementia** may be due to either chronic use or an associated thiamine (vitamin B_1) deficiency.

■ **Pick's Disease** results from frontal and temporal lobe atrophy.

■ **Major Depressive Disorder** can mimic dementia (PSEUDODEMENTIA).

■ **Dementia due to General Medical Conditions** may result from neoplasms, normal pressure hydrocephalus, demyelinating illnesses, trauma, toxic encephalopathies, and infectious diseases (e.g., HIV).

■ **Normal Aging** is associated with minor memory problems (without the impairment of learning) that do not interfere with functioning (BENIGN SENESCENCE).

ID/CC A 63-year-old man is brought to the ER by ambulance after having been found stumbling **drunk** through Times Square.

HPI The patient was admitted to the medical unit for evaluation of **confusion** and **drowsiness that persisted despite resolution of his acute intoxication**. During hospitalization, he could not remember the names of his doctors (ANTEROGRADE AMNESIA) or past events (RETROGRADE AMNESIA) and often **fabricated answers** to questions (CONFABULATION).

PE VS: normal. PE: hepatomegaly; **nystagmus; polyneuropathy**; impaired left lateral gaze (CN VI OPHTHALMOPLEGIA); **ataxia**.

Labs CBC: macrocytic anemia (due to folate deficiency). Lytes/UA: normal. BUN and creatinine within normal limits. LFTs: AST and ALT elevated in a 2:1 ratio. **Serum thiamine pyrophosphate low**.

Imaging CT, head: normal.

Pathogenesis Thiamine deficiency, in this case secondary to chronic alcoholism, is associated with CNS lesions located in the thalamus, hypothalamus, midbrain, pons, medulla, fornix, cerebellum, and mammillary bodies. **Wernicke's encephalopathy** (characterized by **ataxia, ocular abnormalities**, and **confusion**) may progress to **Korsakoff's psychosis** (characterized by **amnesia** and **confabulation**). When both entities exist, a diagnosis of Wernicke–Korsakoff syndrome is made.

Management **Thiamine** (vitamin B_1) IV or PO, administered daily. Since glucose depletes thiamine stores, thiamine administration should always precede glucose. Treatment should be continued for 1 to 2 weeks for Wernicke's encephalopathy and 3 to 12 months for Korsakoff's psychosis. Prompt treatment of Wernicke's encephalopathy may prevent progression to Korsakoff's psychosis. Thiamine replacement may reverse ataxia, ophthalmoplegia, and nystagmus; however, amnesia and confusion do not respond as effectively to treatment, and full recovery of normal cognitive function is rare.

Complications Inadequate or delayed treatment may result in **progressive dementia** and **permanent psychosis**.

Atlas Link ᴜᴄᴠ1 PG-BC-086

Differential Diagnosis ■ **Acute Intoxication** from alcohol or other substances can be associated with the same nonspecific neurologic findings as

Wernicke–Korsakoff syndrome; a careful history along with a toxicology screen are thus essential to diagnosis.

■ **Alcohol Withdrawal** can lead to delirium tremens (delirium, autonomic hyperactivity, and seizures); Wernicke–Korsakoff syndrome is not associated with autonomic instability and may persist despite prolonged abstinence from alcohol.

ID/CC	A 42-year-old **woman** is referred to a psychiatrist for **depressed mood** and inability to seek new employment after having been **fired from her job** 3 months ago.
HPI	Since her dismissal, she has become **withdrawn** and is **overwhelmed** by the thought that no one will hire her. She often **cries** at night, but her **symptoms seem out of proportion to the stress** of having lost her job. On careful screening, she **does not fulfill the criteria for a major depressive episode**.
PE	Physical and neurologic exams within normal limits.
Pathogenesis	Adjustment disorder is caused by an **identifiable stressor** arising against the backdrop of genetic factors, psychosocial factors, and biologic predispositions. Once the stressor is removed, the symptoms do not persist for more than an additional 6 months.
Epidemiology	These disorders are about **twice as common in women** than in men. Individuals with maladaptive stress-coping mechanisms are at increased risk. The prognosis is generally favorable, with > 70% completely recovering by 5 years; comorbid personality disorders or the presence of other psychiatric illnesses worsen the prognosis.
Management	**Psychotherapy** to identify the stressors and develop new stress-coping mechanisms is the treatment of choice. If the patient is refractory to psychotherapy or if depressed/anxious symptoms are prominent, pharmacotherapy should be considered. **Benzodiazepines** (lorazepam, clonazepam, alprazolam) are useful for controlling anxiety, while **antidepressants** (particularly SSRIs) may be helpful for depressive symptoms.
Differential Diagnosis	■ **Major Depressive Disorder** is distinguished from adjustment disorder by the fact that adjustment disorder does not fulfill five of the nine criteria for major depressive disorder (depressed mood, anhedonia, sleep disturbance, appetite change, psychomotor retardation or agitation, feelings of excessive guilt and/or hopelessness, decreased concentration/memory, and morbid preoccupations, including suicidality). In diagnosing adjustment disorder, there must be an identifiable stressor within 3 months of the time that behavioral symptoms arise.

ADJUSTMENT DISORDER

■ **Anxiety Disorders (generalized anxiety disorder, panic disorder, post-traumatic stress disorder)** can be distinguished from adjustment disorder on the basis of symptom quality and severity. Flashbacks, hyperarousal states, and panic attacks generally do not occur in adjustment disorder. The typical initial stressor of post-traumatic stress disorder is a trauma or life event of unusual or catastrophic character.

ID/CC	A 32-year-old woman seeks help because she fears she is "going crazy."
HPI	She lives in New York City and has become increasingly home-bound over the last few months because she **fears going out into public places** such as markets, the subway, and buses. Her **intense anxiety** in various public places has caused her to withdraw from her family and friends (AVOIDANCE OF ANXIETY-PROVOKING SITUATIONS). She reports normal sleep, appetite, and energy levels. There is no past history of traumatic events or obsessive-compulsive behavior.
PE	Physical and neurologic exam normal.
Labs	Lytes/CBC: normal. TFTs: normal. UA: toxicology negative.
Pathogenesis	The etiology of agoraphobia is unknown.
Epidemiology	Prevalence is 1%.
Management	As in panic disorder, antidepressants such as the **tricyclics** (imipramine), **SSRIs** (fluoxetine, fluvoxamine), and **MAO inhibitors** (phenelzine) are useful pharmacologic treatments. **Benzodiazepines** are also effective and provide rapid symptomatic relief in the acute period. **Propranolol** may be used if sympathetic hyperarousal is prominent. **Cognitive behavioral therapy** (CBT) is usually as effective as pharmacotherapy; CBT includes **systematic desensitization**, relaxation techniques, reinterpretation of bodily symptoms, and breathing techniques.
Complications	These patients frequently do not seek medical attention because of their fear of leaving their own homes.
Differential Diagnosis	■ **Panic Disorder with Agoraphobia** describes panic attacks that occur along with a fear of places in which escape would be difficult or a fear that help may not be available if needed.
	■ **Major Depressive Disorder** may result in social withdrawal and anxiety, but the fundamental features are depressed mood, anhedonia, impaired concentration, sleep and weight disturbances, and excessive guilt.

AGORAPHOBIA

■ **Social Phobia** should be diagnosed if the fear of embarrassment and anxiety are directly related to social or performance-related situations.

■ **Specific Phobia** can be differentiated from agoraphobia on the basis of the anxiety-provoking cue; in agoraphobia, the fear is of being in places in which escape is difficult or embarrassing, whereas the anxiety in specific phobia is associated with a particular object or situation.

ID/CC A 29-year-old married **woman** visits her internist because she has been unable to conceive for 3 months.

HPI The patient is **restless and fidgety**, stating that she is worried that she might not be able to have a child. After being offered reassurance, she becomes anxious and indicates that she has felt **on edge** for **at least the last 6 months**. She also admits to being **irritable** and adds that she has had **trouble falling asleep**. She constantly **worries most of the day** about various things, such as whether her husband will leave her, whether something might happen to her mother, and whether her boss will fire her. She states that her worries create **muscle tension** and **impaired concentration**.

PE Physical and neurologic exam normal.

Labs Lytes/CBC: normal. TFTs: normal. UA: toxicology screen negative. ECG: normal.

Pathogenesis Various biologic mechanisms, including the GABA, serotonin, and norepinephrine systems, have been implicated in generalized anxiety disorder (GAD). Psychological factors, including life stressors, strained interpersonal relationships, maladaptive behavioral patterns, and unexpressed impulses/thoughts, are also thought to be important, but it is likely that an interaction between biologic and psychosocial factors leads to the disorder.

Epidemiology Generalized anxiety disorder is a very common condition that is frequently seen by primary care physicians. Prevalence is about 5% in the general population, and the **female-to-male ratio is approximately 2 to 1**. As many as 50% of patients with GAD suffer from a comorbid psychiatric disorder.

Management Psychotherapy, cognitive behavior therapy, relaxation techniques, and lifestyle modification (reduction of caffeine or other stimulant drugs) are useful **psychosocial interventions**. Pharmacologic agents used to treat GAD include **benzodiazepines** (diazepam, lorazepam, alprazolam), **tricyclic antidepressants** (imipramine), and **SSRIs** (sertraline, fluoxetine, paroxetine). Another anxiolytic agent, **buspirone**, is also used effectively as a primary agent. Benzodiazepines provide the quickest onset of symptomatic relief, but continued use beyond 2 to 3 weeks poses a risk of dependence. SSRIs, tricyclic antidepressants, and buspirone may require 1 to 4 weeks of treatment before symptoms significantly improve. A commonly

GENERALIZED ANXIETY DISORDER

used treatment regimen involves administration of benzodiazepines in the acute period; this provides the patient with rapid symptomatic relief while waiting for the therapeutic effect of the SSRIs, tricyclics, or buspirone to take effect. **Beta-blockers** (propranolol) can be helpful in diminishing excess sympathetic outflow (i.e., to relieve palpitations, increased heart rate, and tremor), although typically they are not effective for the full range of anxiety symptoms seen in GAD and are thus best used as an adjunct to more traditional treatments.

Complications

Frequently, patients with GAD initially present to primary care physicians with somatic complaints. Lack of careful attention to chronic feelings of worry and stigmata of anxiety can thus lead to extensive, costly, and perhaps unnecessarily invasive procedures. Up to 50% of patients with an anxiety disorder meet the criteria for a **major depressive disorder**.

Differential Diagnosis

■ **Anxiety Disorder due to General Medical Condition** is diagnosed if patient has a medical condition that results in anxiety; these include pheochromocytoma, hyperthyroidism, paroxysmal tachycardia, carcinoid syndrome, COPD, epilepsy, and hypoglycemia.

■ **Panic Disorder** is characterized by spontaneous episodes of hyperarousal resulting in panic attacks followed by a debilitating fear of recurrent attacks.

■ **Substance-induced Anxiety Disorder** may be precipitated by caffeine, cocaine, thyroxine, alcohol, theophylline, anticholinergics, and corticosteroids.

■ **Hypochondriasis** causes anxiety that is related to a specific fear and preoccupation with having an illness.

■ **Obsessive-Compulsive Disorder** includes intrusive, anxiety-producing thoughts or images (OBSESSIONS) that may lead to compulsive behaviors in which patients engage to lessen the anxiety.

ID/CC	A 28-year-old man presents to the ER worried that his severely chapped hands may have become infected.
HPI	The patient has been **obsessed** with thoughts of infection from contact with the environment and spends **several hours each day scrubbing his hands** with iodine soap to keep them clean. His persistent and **intrusive thoughts** regarding infections are quite **distressing** (EGO DYSTONIC), making it difficult for him to leave his home. The patient also admits to being afraid that his gas stove will accidentally be kept on (OBSESSIONS) and that he will die of asphyxiation during the night; consequently, he **checks his stove 26 times** before going to bed to make certain it is turned off (COMPULSIONS). The patient **acknowledges that his behavior is senseless** but is unable to control it.
PE	Severely desquamated skin with mild bleeding over both hands.
Pathogenesis	Genetic and neurobiologic factors have been implicated in the pathogenesis of obsessive-compulsive disorder (OCD). Structural and neurochemical abnormalities (especially in serotonin transmission) located in the orbitofrontal cortex and basal ganglia have been associated with OCD as well.
Epidemiology	Lifetime prevalence is 2% to 3%; males and females are affected in equal number. It is found in > 10% of psychiatric outpatient clinics. Comorbidity with **major depression** is very high (approximately 60%), and it has also been estimated that 6% to 8% of patients with OCD have **Tourette's disorder**. Interestingly, 30% to 40% of Tourette's disorder patients have OCD symptoms.
Management	First-line medication includes **high-dose SSRIs** (fluoxetine, paroxetine, fluvoxamine, sertraline) and the tricyclic antidepressant **clomipramine** over a period of 16 to 18 weeks. **Behavioral therapy** and psychoeducation are also important in the treatment of OCD. Behavioral therapy involves evoking anxiety associated with fears and obsessions and curtailing subsequent compulsive behaviors. Although unusual, in refractory OCD neurosurgery (cingulotomy, limbic leukotomy, or anterior capsulotomy) may be useful.
Differential Diagnosis	■ **Obsessive-Compulsive Personality Disorder (OCPD)** is associated with chronic, pervasive personality traits such as preoccupation with detail, rigidity, perfectionism, and orderliness; additionally, OCPD lacks the true obsessions or compulsions present in OCD. Patients with OCPD do not feel that their

7 **OBSESSIVE-COMPULSIVE DISORDER**

actions are inconsistent with their overall personality, whereas patients with OCD report that their actions are foreign and distressing.

■ **Psychotic Disorders** such as schizophrenia and delusional disorder are usually not ego dystonic and manifest with specific psychotic symptoms such as delusions, bizarre behavior, or hallucinations.

■ **Anxiety Disorders** can be distinguished from OCD by their lack of specific rituals, obsessions, and compulsions.

■ **Tourette's Disorder** manifests as motor tics that can be difficult to distinguish from the compulsive behavior seen in OCD. Compulsions can be a means of relief from obsessions in patients suffering from OCD, whereas in Tourette's disorder the actions are performed involuntarily.

ID/CC	A 35-year-old **woman** presents to a cardiologist after an episode of **chest pain, palpitations**, and **dizziness**.
HPI	The patient's symptoms arose while she was on a bus going to work this morning and lasted for **less than 10 minutes.** She had two similar episodes while in church that were less severe but sufficiently intense that she **thought she was going to die** (FEELINGS OF IMPENDING DOOM). Since these episodes, she **fears recurrent attacks** and has avoided attending church (CHANGE IN BEHAVIOR DUE TO ATTACKS). Other symptoms that occur during the attacks include **nausea, sweating, tingling sensations** (PARESTHESIAS), **and hot flashes**.
PE	Physical and neurologic exam normal.
Labs	Lytes/CBC: normal. B_{12} and folate: normal; TFTs within normal limits; RPR/VDRL nonreactive. UA: normal; urine toxicology negative; urinary catecholamines normal. ECG: normal sinus rhythm with no evidence of ischemia or infarction.
Pathogenesis	Dysregulation of both central and peripheral (autonomic) nervous systems has been implicated in panic disorder.
Epidemiology	Prevalence is 1% to 3%. **Females** are affected **more often than males** by a ratio of 2 to 1. Average age of onset is 25 (displays a bimodal distribution with peak in late adolescence and another in the mid-30s).
Management	Psychotherapy, cognitive behavior therapy, relaxation techniques, and lifestyle modification (reduction of caffeine or other stimulant drugs) are useful psychosocial interventions. **Cognitive behavioral therapy** has been shown to be as effective as or more effective than pharmacotherapy in the long-term treatment of panic disorder. Antidepressants commonly used in panic disorder include **tricyclic antidepressants** (imipramine, clomipramine), **SSRIs** (sertraline, fluoxetine, paroxetine, citalopram), and **MAO inhibitors** (phenelzine). Treatment with antidepressants may require 1 to 4 weeks before symptoms significantly improve. A commonly used treatment regimen involves administration of **benzodiazepines in the acute period** for rapid symptom relief while waiting for the therapeutic action of the antidepressants. **Beta-blockers** (propranolol) can be helpful in diminishing excess sympathetic outflow (i.e., in relieving palpitations, increased heart rate, tremor) associated with the

PANIC DISORDER WITHOUT AGORAPHOBIA

onset of a panic attack. Pharmacotherapeutic interventions can result in a dramatic decrease in the frequency of panic attacks.

Differential Diagnosis ■ **Anxiety Disorder due to a General Medical Condition** is anxiety caused by medical conditions. Hyperthyroidism, hypoglycemia, pheochromocytoma, cardiac arrhythmias, epilepsy, and hyper-parathyroidism are some common medical disorders that may present with anxiety/panic symptoms.

■ **Post-traumatic Stress Disorder** may have panic attacks that do not occur spontaneously but are related to specific traumatic stimuli or cues.

■ **Specific Phobias** relate to well-delineated objects or situations and do not occur spontaneously.

■ **Panic Disorder with Agoraphobia** describes panic attacks that occur along with a fear of places in which escape would be difficult or a fear that help may not be available if needed.

ID/CC A 21-year-old female college student presents to her primary care physician complaining of **irritability, anxiety, trouble sleeping**, and **difficulty concentrating** (INCREASED AROUSAL).

HPI She reports feeling more **withdrawn** (DETACHMENT) from friends over the past few months and is now starting to miss class regularly. She says she is **fearful** of walking alone through Harvard Square, frequently **avoiding** it altogether, and expresses doubt about whether she'll be able to complete her studies (PERSISTENT AVOIDANCE). Upon further questioning, she reveals that 6 months ago she was **raped** (EVENT) by a male acquaintance while walking across campus. She describes feeling **intense helplessness** and **horror** after the event, although she is **unable to recall specific details**. For **> 1 month**, she has been experiencing horrible **nightmares** and **flashbacks** (INTRUSIVE THOUGHTS) of being sexually assaulted.

PE Patient **hypervigilant** throughout exam and demonstrates an **exaggerated startle reaction** (STATE OF HYPERAROUSAL).

Pathogenesis Post-traumatic stress disorder (PTSD) is defined by its causal origin—that is, there must be a **severe identifiable stressor** that results in its distressing symptomatology. A latency period of months to years may intervene between the trauma and the onset of symptoms. With regard to pathophysiology, alterations in the hypothalamic-pituitary-adrenal axis and increased sympathetic tone have been implicated.

Epidemiology Lifetime prevalence in the community ranges from 1% to 3%. Risk factors for developing PTSD after exposure to a severe stressor include **poor premorbid social supports, younger age, and socioeconomic difficulties**. High-risk populations (rape victims, war veterans, survivors of natural disasters) have higher prevalence rates (14% to 58%). Genetic vulnerabilities and comorbid psychiatric illnesses may predispose one to PTSD. Approximately 30% of patients recover completely; 60% have partial responses to treatment, and 10% either remain the same or worsen. Preexisting or comorbid psychiatric disorders worsen the overall prognosis.

Management **Psychotherapy** is key to long-term recovery. Modalities of therapy include cognitive behavioral therapy, **group therapy**, family therapy, and relaxation training. Pharmacotherapy is used to target prominent symptoms such as depression, anxiety, or intrusive thoughts. Drugs found helpful include **SSRIs** (fluoxetine, sertraline), **tricyclic antidepressants** (amitriptyline,

POST-TRAUMATIC STRESS DISORDER

imipramine), and **MAO inhibitors** (phenelzine). Benzodiazepines (lorazepam, diazepam) may be useful to counter hyperarousal.

Differential Diagnosis

■ **Acute Stress Disorder** is distinguished from PTSD on the basis of the time course of symptoms. Acute stress disorder is diagnosed when symptoms last for a minimum of 2 days and a maximum of 1 month; additionally, the symptoms themselves must occur within 1 month of the traumatic event.

■ **Depression** involves symptoms such as anhedonia, restricted affect, poor concentration, and feelings of detachment, but recurrent and intrusive trauma-related recollections and hypervigilance are not present.

■ **Panic Disorder** may present with autonomic hyperactivity; in PTSD, panic attacks are elicited by trauma-related recollections or cues.

■ **Generalized Anxiety Disorder** and PTSD share similar hyperarousal symptoms, but the latter lacks intrusive symptoms and trauma as the source of concern.

■ **Obsessive-Compulsive Disorder** and PTSD both involve repetitive and intrusive symptoms; if the symptoms can be linked to a traumatic origin, PTSD is the likely diagnosis.

■ **Adjustment Disorder** represents a brief maladaptive response to life stressors that is not associated with the constellation of symptoms seen in PTSD (flashbacks, recurrent dreams, avoidance behavior, numbing, autonomic hyperactivity).

ID/CC	A 23-year-old graduate student in physics experiences **intense anxiety** at research meetings when she is asked to contribute her comments. She also has **excessive fears that she will act in a manner that will be embarrassing** at various social events.
HPI	In addition to anxiety, she experiences **sweating, trembling, and palpitations** during these meetings. She is concerned that she will embarrass herself, although she realizes that her **anxiety is excessive for the situation.** She experiences similar symptoms in other performance situations and at social gatherings.
PE	Physical and neurologic exam normal.
Labs	Lytes/CBC: normal. B_{12} and folate: normal; TFTs: normal; RPR/VDRL nonreactive. UA: normal; toxicology negative.
Pathogenesis	The etiology of social phobia is unknown, but genetic, learning, personality, and biologic factors have been implicated.
Epidemiology	Has a lifetime prevalence of 3% to 13%; onset typically occurs in **adolescence. Females** are affected more frequently than males. The peak age of onset is in the teens.
Management	**SSRIs** and **benzodiazepines** are first-line treatments. **Beta-blockers** (e.g., propranolol) can be used as an adjunct to primary treatments when attendance at social events can be anticipated. **Cognitive behavioral therapy** is effective and includes relaxation strategies, social skills development, cognitive retraining, and desensitization.
Differential Diagnosis	■ **Separation Anxiety Disorder** is seen in children who are reluctant to enter social situations out of a concern for leaving their caretaker; what distinguishes these children from patients with social phobia is that they are comfortable in social situations with their caretaker present.
	■ **Avoidant Personality Disorder** describes a maladaptive and pervasive personality pattern involving an avoidance of interpersonal contact, an unwillingness to get involved with people for fear of being rejected, and a preoccupation with being criticized or feeling inadequate. This diagnosis may coexist with a generalized social phobia and may actually be clinically indistinguishable from social phobias. A careful history of pervasive avoidance of even intimate social contact suggests avoidant personality disorder.

10 **SOCIAL PHOBIA**

■ **Shyness, Stage Fright, or Performance Anxiety** are extremely common but are not associated with the level of clinical distress or the degree of clinical impairment found in social phobia.

■ **Specific Phobia** involves anxiety related to a specific object or situation that does not involve scrutiny, humiliation, or embarrassment. Exposure to the feared stimulus provokes an immediate response.

■ **Panic Disorder with Agoraphobia** describes spontaneous panic attacks that occur along with a fear of places in which escape would be difficult or a fear that help may not be available if needed. These attacks are not limited to social situations.

ID/CC A 6-year-old **boy** is brought to the pediatrician's office for **difficulty organizing tasks, trouble following instructions, forgetting homework assignments**, and **losing things** (SYMPTOMS OF INATTENTION).

HPI He also **makes careless mistakes** in his schoolwork and often **does not seem to listen when spoken to directly**. According to his parents, the patient has always been forgetful and inattentive, but his problems have worsened over the past 6 months and have resulted in **poor grades**. His teachers report that he **fidgets** at his desk and **talks more** than any other student (SYMPTOMS OF HYPERACTIVITY). Classmates are often angry with him because he interrupts others and **blurts out answers** (SYMPTOMS OF IMPULSIVITY). He often leaves his seat in the classroom and runs around excessively.

PE Young boy unable to sit still in chair and rapidly tapping feet together; physical and neurologic exams normal.

Labs EEG: normal.

Imaging PET: normal frontal lobe blood supply.

Pathogenesis No specific cause has been identified; a combination of genetic, neurobiologic (catecholamine and dopaminergic systems; frontal lobe dysfunction), environmental (perinatal/neonatal trauma), and psychosocial factors have been implicated. For the diagnosis of attention-deficit hyperactivity disorder (ADHD), some **symptoms of hyperactivity-impulsivity or inattention must have been present before the age of 7**, and impairment must be present **in two or more settings** (e.g., at home and at school).

Epidemiology **Males** are affected more than females by a ratio of 3 to 1; the prevalence rate is 2% to 8%. Incidence is 3% to 5% per year in schoolchildren. Risk factors include a positive family history for ADHD, family discord, low birth weight, and early brain insults. Without treatment, the course and prognosis of ADHD are poor; it has been estimated that approximately 70% of children diagnosed with ADHD continue to have symptoms into adolescence (this is contrary to the myth that children outgrow ADHD in adolescence). Patients are, in addition, at increased risk for substance abuse later in life. Ten to fifteen percent of adolescents with ADHD have persistent symptoms into adulthood.

ATTENTION-DEFICIT HYPERACTIVITY DISORDER

Management

Treatments include **pharmacologic intervention** and **behavioral therapy. Stimulants (methylphenidate**, dextroamphetamine, pemoline) are the most established pharmacologic treatments, while antidepressants, mood stabilizers, and clonidine have been tried with less success. Patients receiving stimulant therapy may develop **vocal or motor tics**; in such cases, the stimulant should be discontinued immediately.

Differential Diagnosis

■ **Conduct Disorder** and ADHD commonly coexist (40% to 60%); however, in conduct disorder there is a violation of the basic rights of others or of age-appropriate societal norms. If conduct disorder exists alone, attention and cognitive organization should be normal.

■ **Major Depressive Disorder** may mimic the symptoms of ADHD with symptoms of inattention, cognitive dysfunction, and irritability. Careful history should include evaluation for mood changes, neurovegetative symptoms, and suicidality.

■ **Anxiety-related Disorders (generalized anxiety disorder, panic disorder, post-traumatic disorder, simple phobias)** may manifest with symptoms of inattention, hyperactivity, and impulsivity. Anxiety disorders occur comorbidly in 25% of children with ADHD. A careful history and interview can help distinguish worries, fears, phobias, and other symptoms of anxiety disorders from ADHD.

■ **Pervasive Developmental and Learning Disorders** must also be distinguished from ADHD; in ADHD, symptoms of inattention and hyperactivity-impulsivity are not better accounted for by the presence of developmental and learning disorders. Nevertheless, ADHD frequently coexists with learning disorders.

■ **Tourette's Disorder and Obsessive-Compulsive Disorder** have clinical presentations that differ significantly from ADHD, but recent research indicates strong comorbidity and the tendency for these three disorders to be present in familial clusters, perhaps suggesting a genetic tie between the three.

ID/CC   A 5-year-old **boy** is brought to the pediatrician's office by his parents, who are concerned about their son's **lack of friends** and **lack of interest in others** (IMPAIRED SOCIAL INTERACTION).

HPI   **Before age 3** he had been brought to the pediatrician's office numerous times for evaluation of **speech delay** and **odd behaviors** such as rocking and hand twisting (REPETITIVE STEREOTYPED BEHAVIORS). He continued to have difficulties and has been **unable to form appropriate personal attachments**. His eye contact is always poor, and his facial expression appears emotionless (IMPAIRMENT IN NONVERBAL BEHAVIOR). He often repeats what other people say (ECHOLALIA), and his parents report that he doesn't play on his own (LACK OF SPONTANEOUS PLAY), appearing to be interested only in examining umbrellas (ABNORMAL, RESTRICTED INTEREST).

PE   Nonreciprocal facial expression; difficult to engage patient in conversation; behavior notable for **stereotyped movements** such as rocking, hand twisting, and grimacing; rather than play with toys, patient lines them up; IQ 90 with greater impairment in verbal skills than in performance (nonverbal function); normal physical characteristics and neurologic exam.

Labs   Lytes/CBC: normal. TFTs: normal; heavy metal panel negative; hearing test shows no abnormality; chromosomal analysis negative for fragile X syndrome. EEG: no abnormality.

Pathogenesis   No specific cause for autism has been identified, but the etiology is likely multifactorial, with neuroanatomical, infectious, genetic, and perinatal insults implicated. Psychosocial and socioeconomic factors are considered important only in the prognosis.

Epidemiology   Affects 0.05% of children under age 12; **males** are affected **more often than females** by a ratio of 4 to 1. **Onset of symptoms** must be present **before age 3** for the diagnosis of autism.

Management   **Psychoeducation is used for family and patient** to improve social skills and language. **Behavioral therapy** is used to reinforce normal social behaviors. There is no cure, but pharmacology may provide symptomatic relief. **Antipsychotics** are useful in improving learning and reducing hyperactivity/irritability. **SSRIs** are useful in treating obsessive-compulsive features and stereotyped movements.

Complications	Carries a poor prognosis, with < 20% achieving a "borderline normal" life in adulthood.
Differential Diagnosis	■ **Asperger's Syndrome** describes individuals with classic symptoms of autism without significant impairment in language (single words are spoken by age 2, meaningful phrases by age 3). Patients often have "special abilities" with mathematics or memory. Their primary inability lies in socially relating to others. Cognitive ability is intact in patients with Asperger's syndrome.

■ **Rett's Syndrome** involves deceleration of head growth, development of stereotyped hand movements (hand wringing or washing), poorly coordinated gait, impaired social interactions, and impairment in expressive and receptive language. It typically occurs in **girls** between the ages of 5 months and 4 years.

■ **Mental Retardation** is diagnosed when IQ is < 70; it may coexist with autism.

■ **Psychosocial Deprivation** can result in autism-like symptoms but may improve when the environment is corrected.

■ **Medical Conditions** may present with autistic symptoms; these include fragile X syndrome, Down's syndrome, tuberous sclerosis, and phenylketonuria. A thorough medical workup, including brain imaging, genetic analysis, and laboratory examination, is critical in ruling out these medical disorders.

ID/CC	A 10-year-old **girl** is brought to the pediatrician's office as a follow-up visit for pharyngitis.
HPI	Two weeks earlier, the pediatrician recommended fluid and bed rest, as the patient's symptoms appeared viral in origin. Since that time, the patient has noted worsening of her sore throat, difficulty swallowing, and abdominal pain. The mother notes that her daughter has been anxious and irritable and has "not been acting herself." Her attentiveness in school has declined significantly, and she does not want to attend school anymore.
PE	Physical exam significant for erythema of the posterior oropharynx with grayish exudate; abdominal exam normal; neurologic exam normal.
Labs	Lytes/CBC: normal. Throat culture grows *Neisseria gonorrhoeae* on chocolate agar and Thayer-Martin medium.
Pathogenesis	Sexual abuse is **commonly perpetrated by known acquaintances** (e.g., stepfathers, fathers, or other male or female relatives).
Epidemiology	Incidence is 0.25% of children per year; **females are affected more than males**.
Management	**Mandatory reporting** to child protective services followed by appropriate **psychotherapy** for child and family. This applies whenever there is reasonable **suspicion of abuse** even in the presence of denial on the part of the child. Family interventions and establishment of a **safe home environment** are essential to ensuring the safety of the child. Supportive psychotherapy and family therapy will help address the long-term psychosocial sequelae of abuse.
Complications	Sexual abuse as a child has been implicated in the development of **adult psychiatric disorders** such as major depressive disorder, substance abuse, borderline personality disorder, post-traumatic stress disorder, and dissociative disorders.
Differential Diagnosis	■ **Physical Abuse of Children** commonly occurs with sexual abuse. Characteristic signs of physical abuse include cuts or bruises in low-trauma areas (buttocks, genitals, back), burns to the perineum or burns with suspicious patterns (immersion scalding, cigarette marks), multiple fractures of different ages,

spiral fractures of long bones, and retinal hemorrhages ("shaken baby syndrome"). Physical abuse is the leading cause of death in children younger than 1 year.

■ **Physical Neglect** includes signs such as malnutrition, poor hygiene, delayed developmental milestones, and failure to thrive.

ID/CC A **13-year-old boy** is referred to the school psychologist for **repeatedly starting fights** and **stealing** (AGGRESSIVE CONDUCT).

HPI School records reveal increasingly out-of-control behavior for **at least 6 months**. The patient has **run away from home** several times, often **stays out late against parental curfews**, and frequently **misses classes** (SERIOUS VIOLATIONS OF RULES). He has been arrested for vandalism, which has included **setting fires** (DESTRUCTION OF PROPERTY). When interviewed, the patient **denies any wrongdoing** (DECEITFULNESS).

PE Uncooperative, hostile, and provocative when confronted with questions; physical and neurologic exams normal.

Pathogenesis No single identifiable cause of conduct disorder is known. Neurobiologic factors may include catecholamine and serotonin (**low** CSF 5-HIAA) systems.

Epidemiology **Males** are affected **more than females** by a ratio of 4 to 1; the prevalence rate among boys is 6% to 18% in those younger than 18 years. The prevalence of conduct disorder is significantly related to **low socioeconomic status, parental behavioral influence** (antisocial personality disorder, alcoholism), and **the absence of a stable family structure**. Comorbidity with **attention-deficit hyperactivity disorder** (ADHD) and substance abuse is high.

Management Multimodality treatment programs consisting of community and family resources, along with an **environmental structure** with consistent rules and expected consequences. A number of **medications are useful in the treatment of symptoms found in conduct disorder**; among possible treatments are psychostimulants (methylphenidate, dextroamphetamine) for hyperactivity, antidepressants (clomipramine, desipramine, fluoxetine), and α-adrenergic agonists (clonidine). Anticonvulsants (carbamazepine, valproic acid), beta-blockers (propranolol), and neuroleptics (haloperidol, chlorpromazine, risperidone) have also been used to treat various symptoms. Treatment of comorbid disorders such as ADHD, depression, substance abuse syndromes, and learning disorders is important and may help ameliorate the symptoms of conduct disorder.

Complications Conduct disorder predisposes to **antisocial personality disorder**; it is also associated with the triad of enuresis, cruelty to animals, and firesetting.

CONDUCT DISORDER

Differential Diagnosis

■ **ADHD** may complicate the diagnosis of conduct disorder, as there is significant comorbidity with conduct disorder. The clinical focus for ADHD is on attentional disturbances, cognitive dysfunction, and motor hyperactivity.

■ **Depressive Disorders** in children and adolescents often present with atypical symptoms such as agitation, irritability, and disruptive behavior. A careful longitudinal history and assessment of mood can differentiate between depression and the aggressive/destructive behavior of conduct disorder.

■ **Oppositional Defiant Disorder** is distinguished by predominantly negativistic, defiant, and hostile behaviors (patient loses temper, argues with adults, defies adult requests, and blames others for misbehavior). There are no serious violations of social norms or the rights of others.

■ **Substance Abuse Disorder** such as acute alcohol and illicit drug ingestion (cocaine, amphetamines, PCP, marijuana) may produce manifestations of conduct disorder. Careful history and urine toxicology screens are important for an accurate diagnosis.

■ **Learning Disorders** may lead to frustration and disruptive behavior; neuropsychological testing may be used to identify these problem areas.

ID/CC	A **6-year-old** girl is brought to the pediatrician's office after several episodes of **screaming at night**.
HPI	An older sister reports that shortly after falling asleep, the patient sits up in bed **crying** and **appears frightened** while **breathing rapidly and sweating** (AUTONOMIC HYPERAROUSAL). Her sister also notes that although she is **unresponsive to any comforting comments**, the **episodes last no more than 10 minutes**. The patient is **unable to recall any details** of her experience and does not remember it the next morning (AMNESIA). The episodes seem to cluster around periods of increasing stress.
PE	Physical and neurologic exams normal.
Pathogenesis	Sleep terrors are thought to result from **arousal during stages III and IV of non-REM sleep**. Genetic, developmental, and psychological factors are thought to play important roles. Fever, sleep deprivation, and CNS depressants may induce sleep terrors.
Epidemiology	Occurs in 1% to 6% of children but in < 1% of adults. Age of onset is between 4 and 12 years of age in children; the condition **usually resolves spontaneously** during adolescence. In adults, the age of onset is between 20 and 30 years of age.
Management	**Reassurance** that the behavior is usually outgrown by late childhood or adolescence. Security and safety measures are important to protect the individual from injury. The individual **should not be awakened** during an episode of sleep terror or sleepwalking, since this may exacerbate confusion and terror. Pharmacologic management is typically unnecessary, since the behavior often resolves on its own. If sleep terrors are severe, pharmacologic management with **benzodiazepines** (since they suppress stage 4 non-REM sleep, a single bedtime dose provides relief from stage 4 parasomnias) or **imipramine** may prove useful.
Differential Diagnosis	■ **Nightmare Disorder** occurs during REM sleep, and the individual has vivid recollections of the dream. Whereas sleep terrors occur during the first third of the night, nightmare disorder involves the second half of the night and is marked by lack of motor activity, since skeletal muscles are inhibited during REM sleep.
	■ **Sleepwalking Disorder** has a greater degree of organized motor activity, occurs in stages III and IV of non-REM sleep and

SLEEP TERRORS

is not remembered the next morning. Sleepwalking disorder and sleep terrors often coexist.

■ **Seizure Disorders** such as temporal lobe epilepsy may present with stereotyped behavior and postictal confusion; however, incontinence, tonic-clonic movements, and EEG may help identify seizure disorders.

■ **Panic Disorder** patients may awaken at night in a state of fear and hyperarousal; however, the motor hyperactivity and amnesia characteristic of sleep terror are not seen.

ID/CC	A 9-year-old **boy** is brought to the pediatrician's office by his mother because of **uncontrollable, sporadic grunting** (VOCAL TIC).
HPI	The child's mother reports that 4 months ago her son began to utter "bad words" compulsively and could not stop despite admonitions to do so. She denies any history of motor tics but reports that her 16-year-old son is diagnosed with Tourette's syndrome.
PE	Physical and neurologic exams normal.
Pathogenesis	Both genetic and environmental factors play a role in tic disorders, but the mechanism remains unclear.
Epidemiology	The incidence of tic disorders is estimated to be 1 in 100, whereas Tourette's disorder is less common (1 in 2,000); **males are affected more than females by a ratio of 3 to 1.** The mean age of tic onset is 7 years.
Management	**Education** about tic disorders helps patients anticipate symptoms and thus helps reduce frustration. **Behavioral treatments** (habit reversal training, relaxation techniques), individual therapy, and family therapy can be useful to address specific problems that arise. **Dopamine antagonists** (haloperidol, pimozide) are used to suppress tics. Other pharmacologic interventions include **benzodiazepines** (clonazepam, lorazepam) and **α-adrenergic agonists** (clonidine, guanfacine). New atypical neuroleptics (olanzapine, risperidone, quetiapine) may be efficacious; however, studies are lacking. Psychostimulants are frequently used in the treatment of attention-deficit hyperactivity disorder (ADHD) and may exacerbate tic disorders.
Complications	The short-term adverse effects of dopamine antagonists include parkinsonian symptoms, dystonic reactions, and a subjective sense of restlessness (AKATHISIA). The most devastating long-term side effect of treatment with dopamine antagonists is potentially irreversible hyperkinetic movements (TARDIVE DYSKINESIA).
Differential Diagnosis	■ **Tourette's Disorder** must have **both** motor and vocal tics occurring many times a day or intermittently for > 1 year. In contrast, a diagnosis of transient tic disorder requires that motor tics and/or vocal tics be present for > 4 weeks but < 1 year. The onset of tics for both disorders must be before age 18.

TIC DISORDER—TRANSIENT

■ **Chronic Vocal or Motor Tic Disorder** involves either vocal or motor tics (but not both) for > 1 year. To make a diagnosis of transient tic disorder, neither chronic motor or vocal tic disorder nor Tourette's disorder can have been diagnosed in the past.

■ **ADHD** may be comorbid with any of the tic disorders but would be distinguished on the basis of symptoms of hyperactivity and inattention.

■ **Obsessive-Compulsive Disorder** may also coexist with tic disorders; a careful history will aid in diagnosis. Patients would be more likely to have symptoms of persistent and intrusive thoughts that they find distressing.

ID/CC	A 55-year-old **man** is brought to his primary care physician by his daughter following repeated episodes of falling.
HPI	The daughter reports that her father constantly reeks of alcohol. The patient is **annoyed** by **criticism** of his drinking and feels that he drinks only on a social basis. He reports previous unsuccessful attempts to **cut down on his drinking** to prove that he wasn't an alcoholic. At times he admits to **feeling guilty** about his drinking but feels that there is nothing wrong with "a little liquor in the morning" (EYE OPENER) or "a nightcap now and then." The daughter reports that her paternal uncles both passed away from alcoholic cirrhosis (genetic predisposition).
PE	Mild hepatomegaly.
Labs	LFTs: **elevated GGT; AST and ALT elevated** with a ratio of **> 2:1**.
Imaging	CT, abdomen: hepatomegaly with fatty infiltration.
Pathogenesis	The exact mechanism remains unclear. Genetic vulnerability is thought to play an important role in the development of alcohol dependence.
Epidemiology	The lifetime prevalence of alcohol dependence is approximately 8%, and for alcohol abuse it is 5%; **males are affected more than females** by a ratio of 5 to 1.
Management	**Individual** and **group psychotherapy** (such as Alcoholics Anonymous) is vital to sustained abstinence from alcohol use. Other areas of focus in psychotherapy include relapse prevention and motivation enhancement. Psychotherapy should be goal-oriented and should employ behavior modification techniques when possible. Pharmacologic management includes use of **disulfiram (Antabuse), naltrexone**, or psychotropic medications to treat underlying mental illness. Patients should be warned of the serious consequences of using alcohol while taking disulfiram. Naltrexone, an opiate receptor antagonist, is thought to diminish the pleasurable response and internal reward mechanism that is associated with chronic alcohol intoxication.
Complications	Medical complications include alcoholic cirrhosis, pancreatitis, Wernicke–Korsakoff syndrome (a manifestation of thiamine deficiency), alcoholic cardiomyopathy, increased risk of fetal alcohol

ALCOHOLISM

syndrome, aspiration pneumonia, iron and folate deficiency, gastritis, gastric ulcer, varices, cerebellar degeneration, and peripheral neuropathies. When alcohol consumption occurs concomitantly with disulfiram treatment, acetaldehyde levels increase and cause nausea/vomiting, headache, flushing, and tachycardia. Withdrawal is associated (in chronic abusers) with high risk of delirium tremens (including seizures) and should be treated with **benzodiazepines**.

Differential Diagnosis

■ **Alcohol Dependence** requires significant impairment and distress along with at least three of the following symptoms within the last year: tolerance, withdrawal, taking of the substance over a longer period of time or in greater amounts than intended, failure to decrease use, spending a disproportionate amount of time obtaining the substance, reduction or discontinuation of important recreational activity, and use of alcohol in spite of persistent negative physical/psychological consequences.

■ **Alcohol Abuse** requires distress or impairment along with at least one of the following: impairment of major social or occupational role obligations, repeated use in hazardous situations, legal problems resulting from recurrent use, and continued use despite persistent negative interpersonal consequences.

ID/CC A 21-year-old male college student comes to the ER after **smoking marijuana** for the first time.

HPI He denies any loss of consciousness and is alert. He doesn't recall exactly what happened but states that he remembers having felt "unreal," as though he were watching himself from the outside (DEPERSONALIZATION). He denies any hallucinations but does report feeling **anxious** that someone might have been "tailing him" (PARANOID IDEATION). He reports that the 10-minute ride to the hospital "lasted 5 hours" (DISTORTED TIME SENSE) and adds that he was **incredibly hungry** ("MUNCHIES") and had increased sexual desire soon after smoking.

PE VS: **tachycardia** (HR 105). PE: **dry mouth; injected conjunctiva**.

Labs UA: positive for cannabis (will test positive for 7 to 10 days after use or up to 4 weeks in cases of heavy use).

Pathogenesis *Trans*-tetrahydrocannabinol (THC) is the active ingredient in marijuana and acts via the cannabinoid receptor. THC is highly lipophilic, which accounts for the fact that it may be detected up to 4 weeks after ingestion.

Epidemiology Marijuana use has been on the decline since the 1970s, but it is still the **most commonly used "illicit" substance in the world**.

Management **Education** and **psychotherapy** to explore reasons for use. Individual and group psychotherapy may be useful in discussing abstinence issues and relapse prevention. In extreme cases, abstinence can be monitored by urine toxicology.

Complications Motor skills are decreased and judgment may be impaired, but intoxication has minimal direct morbidity and is never fatal. Delirium, psychosis, and anxiety can occur with intoxication. Physiologic withdrawal symptoms are rare (no physical dependence), but psychological dependence is common. Chronic use may be associated with decreased sexual function and amotivational syndrome.

CANNABIS INTOXICATION

ID/CC A **32-year-old man** is brought to the ER complaining of **severe chest pain**.

HPI Upon further questioning, the patient admits that he has been on a **crack cocaine binge**. About 1 month ago he lost his job (FAILURE TO FULFILL MAJOR ROLE OBLIGATIONS) after testing positive for cocaine on a urine toxicology screen; in addition, he was recently arrested on charges of possession (SUBSTANCE-RELATED LEGAL PROBLEMS). He claims to use crack cocaine only on weekends and has a history of fairly long periods of abstinence. He denies requiring escalating doses of cocaine to reach his "high" (LACK OF TOLERANCE).

PE VS: hypertension (BP 168/110); tachycardia (HR 120). PE: dilated pupils (MYDRIASIS).

Labs CBC/Lytes: normal. Troponin I not elevated (rule out MI). ECG: sinus tachycardia with ST depression (evidence of ischemia). UA: urine toxicology remains positive for 1 to 3 days in occasional users and 7 to 12 days in heavy users.

Imaging PET: high activation in the mesolimbic dopamine system.

Pathogenesis The acute behavioral effects of cocaine are related to **dopamine reuptake inhibition**, which results in increased extracellular levels of dopamine in the mesolimbic and mesocortical tracts. The increased dopaminergic transmission in the mesolimbic system may reinforce reward-seeking behavior. Cocaine has also been hypothesized to affect the **serotonin and norepinephrine** system. Peripheral cardiovascular effects are related to reduced norepinephrine reuptake (sympathomimetic action).

Epidemiology The lifetime prevalence of cocaine use is 12%; **males use cocaine more often** than females by a ratio of 4 to 1. The highest frequency of use occurs between the ages of 18 and 25.

Management To obtain abstinence, it is often necessary to institute hospitalization to alter the social and environmental cues that may create craving. **Individual or group psychotherapy** forms the cornerstone of treatment. It is important to **address potential medical complications** of cocaine use in a prompt fashion. Modalities of psychotherapy include relapse prevention therapy, lifestyle modification treatment through group psychotherapy (cognitive behavioral, supportive, etc.), and peer-supervised programs such as a 12-step program. **Pharmacotherapy remains**

experimental, and there is currently no FDA-approved treatment; agents that have been used include dopaminergic agonists (bromocriptine, amantadine), levodopa, mazindol, desipramine, naltrexone, and anticonvulsants.

Complications   Acute cocaine intoxication may result in life-threatening complications such as cardiac **arrhythmias, myocardial infarction, cerebrovascular hemorrhage**, malignant hypertension, and seizure activity.

Differential Diagnosis   ■ **Cocaine Dependence** can be differentiated from cocaine abuse by the degree of social and work impairment, the presence of tolerance, or the occurrence of a withdrawal syndrome when the substance is stopped.

■ **Amphetamine Intoxication** may last from hours to days, whereas the short half-life of cocaine results in a peak effect within 20 minutes.

ID/CC A 52-year-old man who was admitted to the VA hospital for pneumonia complains of **tremor, insomnia**, and seeing "spiders crawling all over the walls" (VISUAL HALLUCINATIONS) after his third hospital day.

HPI The patient is unable to give a coherent history but does indicate that he **stopped drinking alcohol** 4 days ago. Nursing staff indicate that last night he was complaining of feeling **nauseous, sweaty** (DIAPHORESIS), and **anxious**. Tonight he appeared **confused and became agitated** as he accused his nurse of trying to poison him (PARANOID DELUSIONS).

PE VS: **tachycardia** (HR 120); **hypertension** (BP 210/100); tachypnea (RR 22); fever (39.4°C). PE: dilated pupils (due to sympathetic hyperactivity); **hyperreflexia**; bilateral upper extremity **gross tremor**; on mental status exam, patient is **disoriented** to time and place; attention and concentration are significantly impaired and thought processes are incoherent; patient appears to respond to internal stimuli.

Labs Lytes/CBC: normal. BUN and creatinine: normal. LFTs: elevated AST and ALT in 2:1 ratio.

Pathogenesis Alcohol is thought to exert its psychotropic effects by potentiating GABAergic transmission. Cross-tolerance at the GABA receptors occurs between alcohol and benzodiazepines; it is this cross-tolerance that allows benzodiazepines to be used in preventing alcohol-induced withdrawal.

Epidemiology The **mortality rate** of delirium tremens (DTs) has been estimated to be as **high** as 20% if left untreated. Death usually occurs as a result of concomitant systemic medical illnesses. Five percent of all alcoholic patients who are hospitalized have DTs.

Management The mainstay of treatment is **benzodiazepine** administration and taper (to prevent withdrawal symptoms). All benzodiazepines are equally efficacious in preventing alcohol withdrawal; however, oxazepam and lorazepam (Ativan) may be useful in hepatic failure, since their metabolites are readily excreted without extensive liver metabolism. Patients should be well hydrated and given **parenteral thiamine** for 3 to 4 days. **Neuroleptics** may also be used to manage severe agitation or psychosis. **Prophylaxis with anticonvulsants** is used in patients with a history of alcohol withdrawal–induced seizures.

Complications	DTs typically occur 2 to 7 days after the last drink but occasionally may occur as late as 2 weeks afterward. **Alcohol seizures** may occur 6 to 48 hours after decreasing or stopping alcohol intake.
Differential Diagnosis	■ **Substance-induced Psychotic Disorder** may be differentiated from delirium by level of consciousness and toxicology screen.

■ **Acute Substance Intoxication** such as PCP and amphetamine intoxication can present with symptoms of autonomic hyperexcitability and confusion similar to DTs. Breathalyzer and toxicology screen are important in distinguishing between the two.

■ **Sedative/Hypnotic Withdrawal Syndrome** such as that associated with benzodiazepine and barbiturate withdrawal is difficult to distinguish from acute alcohol withdrawal; differentiation can be made via substance abuse history and urine toxicology.

■ **Delirium due to a General Medical Condition** can be distinguished via a thorough history and physical exam, which can help identify underlying medical illnesses (e.g., infections, metabolic abnormalities, stroke, tumor) that cause delirium.

ID/CC	A 34-year-old woman presents to the ER complaining of **nausea**, diarrhea, **vomiting**, and **unsteady gait** (ATAXIA).
HPI	The patient has **a history of bipolar disorder** and has been treated with lithium for the past 10 years. Yesterday she began feeling ill. She notes **blurred vision** and hand **tremor**, adding that she feels more **fatigued** than usual. This morning she felt dizzy and actually fell to the ground.
PE	VS: tachycardia (HR 108); normal RR; orthostatic hypotension (BP 135/80 sitting and 110/70 standing); fever (38.6°C). PE: horizontal **nystagmus; dysarthria**; coarse hand tremors; **hyper-reflexia** of upper and lower extremities; muscle **fasciculations** throughout; impaired finger-to-nose coordination; ataxic gait.
Labs	Lytes/CBC: leukocytosis. Elevated lithium level of 2.5 (therapeutic levels 0.8 to 1.2). ECG: sinus tachycardia with T-wave inversion; regular rhythm with no evidence of ischemic changes.
Imaging	MR, brain: normal.
Management	**Hold lithium** until levels return to within normal limits. If symptoms of intoxication are mild and the lithium level is less than 2.5, administer **IV fluid hydration** with normal saline and correct electrolyte abnormalities as long as there is no evidence of CHF or renal failure. Levels above 2.5, regardless of clinical symptoms, constitute a medical emergency. **Hemodialysis** should be used to rapidly decrease toxic lithium levels; even after dialysis, levels should be closely monitored because of reequilibration from tissues.
Complications	Seizure, coma, nephrogenic diabetes insipidus, rash, acne, psoriasis, cardiac arrhythmias, weight gain and hypothyroidism may result from lithium intoxication; permanent complications of intoxication include cerebellar ataxia and anterograde amnesia.
Differential Diagnosis	■ **Delirium due to Other Substances** must be part of differential diagnosis; toxicology screen is vital to proper diagnosis.

LITHIUM TOXICITY

ID/CC	A **19-year-old white** male is brought to the emergency room by ambulance after jumping out the second-floor window of his fraternity house.
HPI	Fraternity brothers report that the patient appeared to be in a **dreamlike state**, claiming to "hear colors" (SYNESTHESIA) and see kaleidoscopic patterns scroll across the walls (VISUAL HALLUCINATIONS). He appeared **restless** and told everyone that he was going to "fly to the ends of the world." On interview, the patient told the doctor that people were trying to kill him (PARANOIA).
PE	VS: hypertension (BP 170/90); tachycardia (HR 110); tachypnea (RR 32); fever (39°C). PE: diaphoretic and tremulous with mild abrasions throughout extremities; neurologic exam significant for upper and lower extremity **hyperreflexia, lack of coordination, blurred vision**, and **dilated pupils** (MYDRIASIS).
Labs	Lytes/CBC: normal. BUN and creatinine: normal. UA: toxicology negative.
Imaging	CT, spine: negative.
Pathogenesis	LSD is a potent **serotonin agonist** with other poorly understood mechanisms of action, one of which activates the locus ceruleus (responsible for sympathetic output). This mechanism is believed to induce the hallucinogenic and psychedelic properties of LSD, which peak at 2 to 3 hours and last up to 12 hours.
Epidemiology	The age group among which use is most common is 15 to 35. Whites are two times more likely to use LSD than African Americans. Approximately 8% of the population has tried LSD in their lifetime.
Management	The primary treatment approach involves **decreasing sensory input** and keeping the patient safe until drug effects wear off. Assure the patient in a calm manner ("TALKING PATIENT DOWN") that he is safe and that his symptoms are a consequence of LSD. If agitation is severe, treatment with **neuroleptic medications** (haloperidol) may help. If anxiety is a prominent symptom, **benzodiazepines** (lorazepam, diazepam) are modestly efficacious.
Complications	Prolonged psychotic symptoms can sometimes be seen in LSD abuse; however, the relationship between psychotic illnesses (e.g., schizophrenia) and hallucinogen-induced psychosis

remains tenuous and controversial. "Bad trips" are usually panic reactions with psychotic symptoms. Users may also experience "flashbacks"—the reexperiencing of sensations caused by LSD without taking the drug.

Differential Diagnosis

■ **Substances** such as **cocaine, amphetamine, and PCP** as well as **alcohol withdrawal** (delirium tremens) can mimic some of the hallucinogenic properties of LSD. A thorough history, urine toxicology, and physical exam searching for signs of drug use help identify the specific substance.

■ **Psychotic Illnesses** such as **bipolar disorder, schizophrenia, and severe depression** are often difficult to distinguish from substance-induced psychosis. The former tends to demonstrate auditory hallucinations, while the latter more often manifests visual symptoms.

ID/CC	A 55-year-old white female with treatment-refractory depression presents to the emergency department complaining of **throbbing headache, diaphoresis**, **anxiety, nausea, vomiting**, and **confusion**.
HPI	She reports that over the past few years she has been placed on numerous antidepressants without success and was recently started on **phenelzine**. She was in her normal state of health until last evening, when she went out to a dinner party with friends. She reports that all she had was some bread, a glass of Chianti **wine**, and a few servings of aged cheddar **cheese**.
PE	VS: **hypertension** (BP 200/120); tachypnea (RR 28); **tachycardia** (HR 124); fever (39.4°C). PE: neurologic exam reveals pupils 6 mm (MYDRIASIS) bilaterally and moderate **muscle fasciculations** throughout; neurologic exam otherwise normal.
Labs	ECG: sinus tachycardia. Lytes/CBC: normal. BUN and creatinine normal. UA: urine toxicology negative.
Imaging	CT, head: normal.
Pathogenesis	Tyramine hypertensive crisis occurs with concomitant use of **MAO inhibitors (phenelzine and tranylcypromine)** and **tyramine-rich products**. The metabolism of tyramine-containing foods is blocked by the inhibition of monoamine oxidase, and the subsequent increase in circulating tyramine leads to the synaptic release of norepinephrine, resulting in a **hyperadrenergic state**. Note that hypertensive crises are more common with MAO-A inhibitors (i.e., phenelzine and tranylcypromine) than with MAO-B inhibitors (selegiline).
Epidemiology	Tyramine-rich foods include aged cheese products, fermented meats (sausage, salami), wine, beer, pickled herring, yogurt, beans, and yeast extracts. Adverse reactions may also occur with concomitant use of MAO inhibitors and sympathomimetics (dopamine, stimulants, decongestants) or serotonergic agents (fluoxetine, sertraline, paroxetine, clomipramine); other potentially fatal interactions occur with meperidine, oral hypoglycemics, and tricyclic antidepressants.
Management	**Discontinue MAO inhibitors**. ABCs and close vital sign monitoring. Pharmacologic management varies depending on severity of hypertension. For mild to moderate hypertensive reactions, **sublingual calcium channel blockers** (e.g., nifedipine 10 to 20 mg) can

be used; more severe cases warrant **IV phentolamine** (α-adrenergic antagonist) or sodium nitroprusside. Beta-blockers should be avoided because they may result in unopposed α-mediated vasoconstriction and may worsen hypertension. When starting an MAO inhibitor, a washout period from other antidepressants of at least 2 weeks is recommended to prevent potentially serious adverse reactions. Drugs with longer elimination half-lives require increased washout periods (e.g., a 6-week washout period for fluoxetine because of its long half-life). **Avoid tyramine-rich foods**.

Complications

Hyperadrenergic crisis may result in potentially fatal complications such as stroke, myocardial infarction, and arrhythmias; therefore, close cardiac and neurologic monitoring is necessary. Patient dietary education is the primary means of preventing this potentially lethal interaction.

Differential Diagnosis

■ **Other Causes of Hypertension** include uncontrolled primary hypertension, pheochromocytoma, thoracic aortic dissection, neuroleptic malignant syndrome, and serotonin syndrome. A careful food and drug history is essential in making the diagnosis.

ID/CC	A 28-year-old man was admitted for observation after being involved in a motor vehicle accident; urine toxicology at admission is positive for opiates.
HPI	On hospital day one, the patient complained of **muscle aches** (MYALGIA), **nausea, runny nose** (RHINORRHEA), **and tearing eyes** (LACRIMATION). On the following day, he became **diaphoretic** and **restless**, demanding to leave the hospital. On day three, the patient **vomited**, soiled his pants with uncontrollable **diarrhea**, and appeared **anxious**.
PE	VS: **fever** (39.6°C); **hypertension** (BP 160/100); **tachycardia** (HR 104); tachypnea (RR 22). PE: **pupillary dilatation** (MYDRIASIS) and **"gooseflesh" skin** (PILOERECTION); multiple punctate lesions or "tracks" seen on patient's forearms, indicating where he had been injecting.
Labs	Normal.
Pathogenesis	In addition to binding readily to primary opiate receptors, opiates suppress adrenergic function in the locus ceruleus. Consequently, opiate withdrawal is characterized by sympathetic hyperactivity. Acute withdrawal symptoms begin approximately 8 hours after the last use, peak in 2 to 3 days, and may last up to 10 days. Some symptoms, such as insomnia, bradycardia, temperature dysregulation, and craving, can persist for up to 6 months following discontinuation.
Epidemiology	Estimates suggest a lifetime prevalence of opiate dependence or abuse of approximately 1.3%, although this number varies across different cultures.
Management	Initial **management is supportive** and focuses on making the patient comfortable. **Methadone**, a long-acting oral opioid, has cross-tolerance with heroin and is often used for both short- and long-term detoxification. **Clonidine**, an α_2-adrenergic agonist, suppresses the autonomic hyperactivity often seen in opiate withdrawal. Careful monitoring of blood pressure for hypotension is indicated when clonidine treatment is first utilized. **Treat comorbid depressive and anxiety symptoms** that are seen in up to 90% of patients with opioid dependence.
Complications	Opiate withdrawal **is not life-threatening**.

OPIATE WITHDRAWAL

Differential Diagnosis ■ A thorough medical and substance abuse history, physical exam, and urine toxicology screen will help distinguish opiate withdrawal from more immediately threatening medical conditions or from withdrawal syndromes due to other substances that may be potentially serious.

ID/CC	A **25-year-old male city dweller** is brought to the emergency department after shouting out obscenities in public and **violently assaulting** a police officer (BELLIGERENCE).
HPI	Neighbors report that the patient had a party last night and suspect he was drinking alcohol. This morning he appeared **agitated** and was knocking on residents' doors shouting, "Stop watching me, you pigs; you've ruined my life" (PARANOID DELUSIONS). Several officers were called in to restrain him.
PE	VS: hypertension (BP 170/100); tachypnea (RR 32); tachycardia (HR 126); fever (38.6°C). PE: neurologic exam reveals vertical and horizontal **nystagmus, unsteady gait** (ATAXIA), slurred speech (DYSARTHRIA), **diminished responsiveness to pain** and **numbness** in upper and lower extremities, increased DTRs (HYPERREFLEXIA), and generalized **muscular rigidity**; mental status exam reveals diffuse **impairments in concentration, memory, and orientation**.
Labs	Lytes/CBC: normal. **Elevated serum CPK** (2,000). UA: positive for **myoglobinuria; urine toxicology positive for PCP**.
Pathogenesis	Psychiatric symptoms are thought to result from antagonism at the PCP receptor site located on the ion-channel-gated **NMDA receptor complex**.
Epidemiology	The highest incidence of PCP intoxication is in men aged 20 to 40. Other risk factors include living in an urban environment and having limited economic and social resources.
Management	ABCs and vital sign monitoring every 2 to 4 hours. **Activated charcoal** and **gastric lavage** if indicated. Agitation can be controlled by **benzodiazepines** (lorazepam, clonazepam, diazepam), while more severe presentations with psychotic symptoms can be managed with **neuroleptics**; care should be taken when using neuroleptics due to the possibility of decreasing the seizure threshold.
Complications	Potentially fatal complications include hypertensive crisis, respiratory arrest, malignant hyperthermia, status epilepticus, and acute renal failure secondary to **rhabdomyolysis** and **myoglobinuria**.

PCP INTOXICATION

Differential Diagnosis

■ **Substances** such as cocaine, amphetamine, and alcohol can mimic PCP psychosis. A thorough history, urine toxicology, and physical exam searching for signs of illicit drug use (septum erosion, needle tracks) help identify the specific substance.

■ **Psychotic Illnesses** such as bipolar disorder, schizophrenia, and severe depression are often indistinguishable from substance-induced psychosis. Although substance abuse may occur comorbidly with major psychiatric illnesses, careful longitudinal history, urine toxicology, and physical exam are key factors in their differentiation. There must be evidence of psychiatric symptoms during extended sobriety for a non-substance-use diagnosis to be made.

ID/CC	A 37-year-old **woman** with chronic schizophrenia, undifferentiated type, is noted by her psychiatrist to **involuntarily pucker her lips** (LIP SMACKING) and make **facial grimaces**.
HPI	A review of the patient's medical records reveals that she was diagnosed with **schizophrenia** 20 years ago and has been treated with a variety of typical **neuroleptic medications** over that period. She is currently on haloperidol 10 mg twice a day and benztropine 1 mg once a day with excellent control of her hallucinations and paranoid delusions.
PE	Neurologic exam significant for **rapid jerking movements** of her shoulders with bilateral upper extremity tremor; **involuntary writhing movements of tongue**.
Labs	Lytes/CBC: normal. TFTs: normal; RPR/VDRL nonreactive.
Imaging	CT, head (noncontrast): normal.
Pathogenesis	The precise cause of tardive dyskinesia (TD) is unknown; however, neuroleptics have been postulated to increase dopamine receptor sensitivity in the striatum and produce neuron-damaging free radicals. TD does not always improve with discontinuation of neuroleptics.
Epidemiology	The risk of TD **increases with the duration of antipsychotic use** (*tardive* means late-appearing) at a rate of **3% to 5% per year**. **Increasing age** (i.e., the elderly) is the greatest risk factor for TD. Other factors that may increase risk include female gender, the presence of a mood disorder, and diabetes mellitus.
Management	After adequate risk/benefit assessment, a decision must be made to **continue the antipsychotics** despite the TD, to **discontinue the antipsychotic**, or to **switch to another neuroleptic**. If the decision is made to continue the current medication, **dose reduction or adjunctive therapy** (vitamin E, beta-blockers, clonidine, benzodiazepines) may be useful. When a decision is made to discontinue the neuroleptic, a slow taper is indicated, with careful monitoring for emergent psychotic symptoms. **During the early phase of the taper, TD may actually worsen before it begins to improve.** Switching to atypical antipsychotic agents such as olanzapine or risperidone may prove useful in the treatment of TD while continuing to control psychotic symptoms. Clozapine may also be used, although on rare occasions it may cause agranulocytosis. If possible, most patients with newly

diagnosed psychotic disorders should be treated with olanzapine, quetiapine, risperidone, or clozapine because of the significantly lower risk for TD.

Complications Severe TD may result in respiratory distress, pronounced dysarthria, dysphagia, and other debilitating neurologic abnormalities. TD is also potentially **socially devastating**, since patients can display strange facial movements throughout the day.

ID/CC A **17-year-old girl** presents to her gynecologist after **missing her last six periods** (AMENORRHEA). She also reports being unable to tolerate the cold weather in Massachusetts and thinks she is **losing her hair**.

HPI She reports feeling **anxious about her weight** and **believes she is fat** (DISTORTED BODY IMAGE). She has been **dieting** and **exercising for several hours a day**. Her parents, both of whom are successful attorneys, have been criticizing her decision to drop out of school to pursue a career in modeling.

PE VS: hypothermia (35.6°C); bradycardia (HR 52); mild hypotension (BP 105/66); height 170 cm (67 in.); weight 41.7 kg (92 lb) (**< 85% of ideal body weight**). PE: thin, emaciated young female; skin dry and scaly with lanugo body hair ("BABY HAIR"); slight pedal edema (HYPOALBUMINEMIA); neurologic exam normal.

Labs CBC: anemia; leukopenia. Lytes: hypokalemia. Hypoalbuminemia; elevated serum β-carotene.

Pathogenesis The etiology of anorexia nervosa is thought to be multifactorial, involving an interplay between predisposing factors (genetic vulnerability, female gender, obsessional characteristics), cultural factors, acute precipitating stressors, and maladaptive behavioral/psychological patterns.

Epidemiology Prevalence is estimated at 0.5%. The average **age at onset is between 13 and 18**. Occurs more commonly in developed countries, among middle- and upper-class Caucasian women, and in professions such as fashion modeling and ballet dancing. **Females** are affected more than males (15:1).

Management **Supportive measures** for possible electrolyte disturbances, nutritional deficiency, cardiovascular compromise, and renal insufficiency. **Hospitalization** is indicated in patients with significant metabolic derangements (hypokalemia, alkalosis, hyponatremia, elevated BUN/creatinine, hypochloremia), cardiac arrhythmias, or body weight below the 75th percentile. **Cognitive behavioral interventions** are the mainstay of treatment. **Family therapy** is the most effective form of psychotherapy; **group therapy** is also useful. Close supervision of caloric intake is an important part of the treatment approach and is often reinforced with behavioral incentives. If patients fail to gain weight, they are placed on bed rest, and **tube feeding** may be necessary if weight remains

ANOREXIA NERVOSA

dangerously low. The efficacy of pharmacotherapy is controversial, but agents that affect the serotonin system (**SSRIs**) are favored and are used to treat the depressive symptoms patients with anorexia nervosa typically experience.

Complications
Hypothermia, fluid/electrolyte abnormalities, edema, osteoporosis, diminished thyroxine levels, hypocortisolemia, decreased estrogen and testosterone, anemia, leukopenia, hypotension, bradycardia, other cardiac arrhythmias, and death (10% to 20% of hospitalized patients die within 10 to 30 years).

Differential Diagnosis
■ **Bulimia Nervosa** can be distinguished from anorexia based on the patient's ideal body weight; in anorexia nervosa, weight is below the 85th percentile. Although bingeing and purging are commonly associated with bulimia nervosa, they can also be features of anorexia and, when present, should be diagnosed as anorexia nervosa, binge-eating/purging type.

■ **Major Depression, Anxiety Disorders** and **Body Dysmorphic Disorder** may have features of distorted body image but are easily distinguished from anorexia nervosa on the basis of body weight and the presence of maladaptive eating/exercising behaviors.

ID/CC A **17-year-old girl** is brought to a psychiatrist by her parents for **worsening self-esteem** and **repeated attempts at "fad diets"**.

HPI When interviewed alone, the girl confides that her troubles started when she entered high school and became self-conscious about her weight. She now sneaks into the kitchen to **consume a tremendous amount of food** in what is usually a **short period of time**. She feels as though she **loses control of her eating** during these episodes. Afterward, she feels disgusted with herself and **induces vomiting** by sticking her fingers down her throat. At times she has "felt depressed" after vomiting but has not had any changes in sleep, energy, interest, or concentration. This behavior has persisted **at least twice a week for 3 months**.

PE **Ragged and worn-appearing enamel** over front teeth; bilaterally enlarged parotid glands on palpation; extremities notable for multiple callus formation on backs of hands and knuckles.

Labs Lytes: hypokalemia; hypochloremia. ABGs: bicarbonate elevated (36 mEq/L). CBC: normal. BUN, creatinine, B_{12}, folate, and TFTs: normal; RPR/VDRL nonreactive.

Pathogenesis Psychological theories regarding the cause of bulimia nervosa include developmental arrest, familial conflict, and pressure to be thin secondary to societal factors. No definite etiology has been identified, although the norepinephrine and serotonin systems have been implicated.

Epidemiology Average age of onset is 13 to 18 years; affects approximately 1% to 3% of women. Prognosis is better than that of anorexia. **Females** are affected more than males (10:1).

Management Even in the absence of a major depressive episode, **antidepressants** are the mainstay of pharmacologic treatment. SSRIs (sertraline, fluoxetine), tricyclic agents (imipramine, desipramine, amitriptyline), and MAO inhibitors (phenelzine, tranylcypromine) have been shown to be effective, although MAO inhibitors have a risk of producing hypertensive crisis. Various **psychotherapeutic modalities** (e.g., cognitive behavioral therapy, interpersonal psychotherapy, psychodynamic therapy, and family psychotherapy) have also been shown to be useful in the treatment of bulimia. **Hospitalization** is necessary in cases of severe electrolyte disturbance or other medical complications associated with bulimia.

Complications Medical complications include dental caries, hypokalemia, metabolic alkalosis, esophagitis, Mallory-Weiss tear, and arrhythmias.

Differential Diagnosis ■ **Bulimia Nervosa, Nonpurging Type** meets the criteria of bulimia nervosa without purging behavior such as self-induced vomiting, laxative abuse, or enema use. The nonpurging type is typically associated with behaviors such as excessive exercise or restricted food intake.

■ **Anorexia Nervosa** can be distinguished from bulimia based on weight. In anorexia, the patient's weight must be < 85% of that expected for age and height.

ID/CC   A 72-year-old man with **progressive dementia** who has been **unable to communicate** for a year is discovered on exam to have colon cancer. He is admitted to the hospital.

HPI   The admitting resident, in clarifying the standing orders for resuscitation (CODE STATUS), takes the initiative to discuss with the patient and family whether an advance directive exists.

Management   An advance directive or power of attorney (DESIGNATED SURROGATE DECISION MAKER) should be consulted in all nonemergency situations before any treatment is initiated in adults **incapable of informed consent**. In the absence of a preexisting document, the determination of mental incompetency to provide informed consent should involve a psychiatric consultation and, if possible, a consultation with a hospital's legal counsel or committee if one exists. An advance directive often specifies a surrogate decision maker, but if it does not do so, the family and/or close associates should be consulted. If there is not an available surrogate or if the surrogates cannot agree on treatment, review by an ethics or judiciary committee should be sought. Ethics committees are also consulted when the surrogate decision is clearly unreasonable or is not based on the patient's previous wishes.

ID/CC A 14-year-old girl is brought to the family physician by her mother for evaluation of a lack of menstrual periods for the past 2 months; in the course of the evaluation she is found to have a positive pregnancy test.

HPI The patient asks the physician not to inform her mother of the results of the test. Later, the mother calls to ask if her daughter is pregnant.

PE Pelvic exam normal.

Labs Positive β-hCG.

Management The patient's confidentiality should be respected; however, disclosure to the parents by the minor should be encouraged. According to the AMA Code of Ethics, when a **minor (age < 18) seeks medical services, confidentiality should be maintained except when state law requires otherwise** (e.g., abortion in some states). Classic cases in which **confidentiality should be maintained include treatment for contraception, STDs, substance abuse, mental illness**, and **pregnancy**. It is, however, recommended that physicians explore the reasons for nondisclosure and facilitate problem solving. It is important to note that confidentiality should be broken to prevent serious harm to the minor or when parental involvement is necessary for treatment decisions. If sexual abuse is suspected, physicians are legally required to report to an appropriate protective agency (not to the parents). Sometimes such situations are ambiguous and require that the physician weigh and balance conflicting duties. Most hospitals have an ethics committee in which such quandaries can be discussed without revealing the identity of the patient. This resource can be helpful in making more informed and thoughtful choices in a difficult situation.

ID/CC A 32-year-old HIV-positive woman, now 24 weeks' pregnant, stopped taking AZT because it made her feel nauseous. Her physician is unsure whether this represents neglect and asks for a psychiatry consult.

HPI Although the patient is informed that taking the medication can reduce the risk of HIV transmission to the fetus from 24% to 8%, she continues to refuse to take the medication.

Management Respect the patient's wishes. Cases involving withholding treatment that would affect a fetus (and not a newborn) do not constitute child abuse in the current U.S. legal system; hence, the wishes of the mother must be respected. As in this case, obtain a psychiatry consult to evaluate competence and/or to explore the mother's thinking. Her fear and confusion merit psychotherapeutic support, and she may change her mind in the context of an alliance that clarifies her thinking.

ID/CC A 24-year-old man with renal failure due to diabetic nephropathy has been doing well on dialysis for 6 months while awaiting an organ donor.

HPI He now wishes to discontinue treatment despite his understanding that he will die without it. Although a psychiatric interview reveals no evidence of a mood or thought disorder, the patient's wife and mother request that dialysis be continued.

Management Respect the patient's wishes. In this case, the patient is a **competent adult** and is able to decide which treatment to accept or deny. It is important to note that the **AMA Code of Ethics does not recognize an ethical distinction between withholding** (never starting) **treatment and withdrawing treatment** (stopping in the middle). The law does, however, distinguish between withholding/withdrawing treatment (which is acceptable) and providing medications to help a terminally ill patient hasten death (which is actionable). Finally, a clinician who respects the patient's wish to die should attend to comfort care (PALLIATION) and affirm the dying process.

ID/CC	A 32-year-old female surgeon is treated for a gunshot wound in the same hospital in which she is completing her residency.
HPI	Later, the chief resident in charge of the call schedule asks the attending physician if he can look at her chart to ascertain when she will recover.
Management	Do not disclose confidential patient records without patient consent. Aspects of patient care should be discussed only with those who are directly involved in that case, not with friends, relatives, or business associates. If confidentiality **is** breached, it is the duty of the physician to inform the patient.

ID/CC   A college student is referred to the psychiatry department by his primary care doctor after reporting that he was turned down by his political science instructor, stating, "If I can't have her no one will; I'm going to kill her."

HPI   While awaiting transfer to the Behavioral Crisis Center, the patient disappears and the doctor is unable to locate him.

Management   Steps required of the physician by law in order to protect potential victims include warning the potential victim and notifying the police or detaining the patient via commitment procedures. This duty is described in the precedent-setting case of *Tarasoff vs. Regents of the University of California*, 551 P.2d 334 (1976). **There is no doctor-patient confidentiality standard that supersedes the duty to report imposed by the Tarasoff ruling**.

ID/CC A neonate with Down's syndrome is born with duodenal atresia.

HPI Although the parents are told that the atresia is surgically correctable and that the newborn will die without treatment, they request that treatment be withheld.

Management Do not withhold treatment. According to the AMA Code of Ethics, treatment **decisions must be made in the neonate's or child's best interests** rather than being based on the desires of the parents. Treatment can be withheld or withdrawn when there is little potential for success, when the risks outweigh the benefits, and when treatment will only extend the child's life such that the pain will exceed any possibilities for a meaningful existence. Note that **withholding of treatment is a form of neglect** that mandates reporting to social services (as for child abuse). Consult psychiatry to evaluate competence and/or to support the parents' psychosocial needs. Maintain a therapeutic alliance in efforts to address their concerns in caring for a child with Down's syndrome. Educate the parents and help them adapt.

WITHHOLDING TREATMENT

ID/CC	A 26-year-old **man** with a history of **unexplained hypoglycemia** presents with weakness and confusion.
HPI	No information is available on three previous episodes of hypoglycemia because they all occurred at other hospitals. He is currently employed as a **nurse's aide** and lives with his sister, who has insulin-dependent diabetes. Five years ago he had an exploratory laparotomy for abdominal pain; a normal appendix was removed at that time.
PE	VS: fever (38°C); tachycardia (HR 105); tachypnea (RR 22). PE: tremor; diaphoresis; diffuse abdominal tenderness.
Labs	Glucose low (25 mg/dL); elevated serum insulin (95 (U/mL) with **decreased C-peptide** ($<$ 0.4 ng/mL); **insulin antibodies present** (indicates exogenous insulin).
Pathogenesis	Psychodynamic theories cite **assumption of the sick role** as the primary motive for factitious disorder. No apparent secondary gain is involved.
Epidemiology	Limited information is available, but factitious disorder has been estimated to account for up to 6% of hospital admissions. **Health care workers** are at increased risk; **males** are affected more than females.
Management	Supportive, **nonaccusatory,** and **empathic confrontation** is often employed. Long-term psychotherapy may be used but is of limited success. No pharmacotherapy has been proven useful.
Complications	Unnecessary medical evaluations and procedures can account for significant morbidity and waste of health care funds. Careful documentation and effective coordination between health care providers may reduce these complications. If the patient is a child and the illness is forcibly inflicted upon them by an adult (MUNCHAUSEN'S SYNDROME BY PROXY), legal intervention and protection of the child is warranted.
Differential Diagnosis	■ **Malingering** also involves symptoms that are feigned, but there is secondary gain (e.g., money, avoiding legal perils) other than assuming the sick role. ■ **Somatoform Disorders** are characterized by symptoms that are not intentionally produced.

ID/CC   A 31-year-old man is seen for evaluation of recent memory problems.

HPI   Four months ago, a 2×4 piece of wood fell off a high shelf at a hardware store, striking the patient. According to ER records, the patient's **mental status exam was normal and the patient denied losing consciousness**. His physical exam was also normal, without evidence of external trauma. He was monitored in the ER and was discharged. However, the patient asserts that since his injury he has **intermittently forgotten** his name and where he is; furthermore, he reports difficulty remembering how to perform his job. He recently **filed for disability** and now **asks for a medical report documenting his disability**.

PE   **Physical and neurologic exam normal**; on mental status exam, patient is alert and oriented to place and time; however, he has difficulty recalling his middle name; patient performs serial sevens with approximate errors (MANIFESTATION OF GANSER'S SYNDROME); short-term memory intact, but patient exhibits defects in remote memories (e.g., date of high school graduation, past presidents).

Labs   Lytes/CBC: normal. TFTs: normal; RPR/VDRL nonreactive; B_{12} and folate: normal.

Imaging   MR, head: normal.

Pathogenesis   The etiology of malingering is based on motivation by an **external gain** (e.g., financial remuneration, legal incentives, evading work/punishment/combat).

Epidemiology   Most commonly occurs in medicolegal cases, in **disability claims**, and among prisoners and military personnel.

Management   **Thorough medical and psychiatric evaluation**. The patient should be given the benefit of the doubt before a diagnosis is established. Once the diagnosis is made, recommendations to the patient should be clearly and consistently articulated. The patient should also be allowed to give up symptoms without losing dignity.

Differential Diagnosis   ■ **True Memory Impairment** following head injury is rare without loss of consciousness and most likely involves amnesia for the accident and for the events leading up to it. Long-term memories are least likely to be affected by mild traumatic injury;

furthermore, loss of orientation to person without other memory deficits seldom occurs. Exaggeration of symptoms on exam is suggestive of malingering or factitious disorder but not true memory impairment.

■ **Factitious Disorder** can be distinguished from malingering based on the nature of the incentive. In factitious disorder, the gain is motivated solely by assumption of the sick role (INTERNAL OR PRIMARY GAIN).

ID/CC	An 18-year-old **man** presents for an evaluation of mental status in preparation for **partial sex-reassignment surgery**.
HPI	The patient states that as far back as he can remember, he has insisted that he is "a woman in a man's body" (INSISTENCE OF CROSS-SEX IDENTITY). He recalls dressing as a girl since the age of 6 (PREFERENCE FOR CROSS-SEX ROLES) and playing with his sister's toys (PREFERENCE FOR STEREOTYPICAL GAMES OF THE OPPOSITE SEX). His parents also report that all of his friends were girls (PREFERENCE FOR OPPOSITE-SEX PLAYMATES) and that he often found little in common with other boys.
PE	Young-appearing male with feminine mannerisms; **normal male genitalia**.
Labs	Karyotype: normal male genotype (**XY**).
Pathogenesis	Psychological factors are considered more important than hormonal factors in the development of gender identity.
Epidemiology	The precise etiology is unknown. This clinical entity is found much **more commonly in biological males** than in biological females. Genetic, hormonal, brain architecture, social learning, and psychoanalytic theories have been advanced in attempts to explain gender identity.
Management	Initial management involves a thorough history, physical examination, and laboratory workup (including **karyotype analysis** in cases where genitalia are ambiguous). **Psychotherapy** is useful for discussing family and other interpersonal issues regarding cross-gender preference. More specifically, psychotherapy may help the patient cope with the stress associated with cross-gender living or offer support/consultation regarding hormone therapy versus sex reassignment. **Group therapy** is useful for diminishing social withdrawal and allows participants to share ideas regarding cultural acceptance. **Sex-reassignment surgery** is used only for adults diagnosed with true gender identity disorder. In these cases, a trial of cross-gender living followed by hormone replacement is indicated before proceeding to surgery.
Complications	Comorbid psychiatric disorders include substance abuse or dependence, anxiety disorders, and depressive disorders.

Differential Diagnosis

■ **Transvestite Fetishism** involves cross-dressing behavior for sexual excitement (most typically occurs in heterosexual men). There is, however, no insistence on cross-sex identity and no desire for sex reassignment.

■ **Normal Variants of Accepted Sexual Behavior** include homo-erotic play, masturbation, and sexual fantasies.

■ **Paraphilias (or abnormal sexual behaviors)** include pedophilia (sexual activity with prepubescent children), exhibitionism (gain of sexual pleasure from publicly displaying genitalia), voyeurism (pleasure from viewing individuals in sexually compromising situations), frotteurism (rubbing or touching nonconsenting persons), sadism (sexual gratification derived from the suffering of the victim), masochism (pleasure from being abused), and fetishism (object of desire is inanimate).

ID/CC A 68-year-old man is less talkative than usual while having his routine physical examination. Upon further questioning, the patient tells his doctor that his **wife passed away 1 month ago** and that he hasn't felt the same since that time.

HPI The patient says he has been **unhappy most of the time** (DEPRESSED MOOD) since his wife's death and hasn't been interested in his usual hobbies (ANHEDONIA). He often wakes up at night and frequently cries when he thinks of his loss.

PE Physical and neurologic examinations normal.

Labs Lytes/CBC: normal. TFTs: normal; RPR/VDRL nonreactive. UA: toxicology screen negative.

Pathogenesis Bereavement is an **appropriate response to the death of a loved one**. If the symptoms of bereavement become severe enough or last longer than cultural norms allow, a diagnosis of major depression must be considered; this phenomenon may also be referred to as pathologic grief or complicated bereavement. Uncomplicated bereavement depression typically begins within 2 months of a death and resolves within 2 months of its onset. The biologic mechanism of complicated bereavement is thought to be similar to that of major depression.

Epidemiology Studies suggest that up to 30% of individuals with bereavement depression eventually develop a formal depressive disorder.

Management **Supportive psychotherapy** is useful to help the patient with feelings of anguish, despair, and loss. If insomnia is prominent, **trazodone, zolpidem**, or **benzodiazepines** can be helpful. For those patients who go on to develop a major depressive disorder, intensive psychotherapy and treatment with **antidepressant medications** are indicated.

Complications Unresolved grief may progress to a **major depressive disorder**.

Differential Diagnosis ■ **Major Depressive Disorder** may be diagnosed if depressive symptoms are severe (i.e., involve morbid guilt, suicidal ideation, feelings of profound worthlessness, frank psychotic features, or significant functional impairment) or if symptoms persist longer

BEREAVEMENT

than currently accepted cultural norms (> 2 months). In bereavement, symptoms are often related to triggers regarding memories of the deceased; this differs from major depression, where symptoms tend to be chronic and recurrent in nature without a specific trigger.

ID/CC	A **30-year-old** man is brought to the hospital by the Los Angeles police after shouting at staff in the lobby of the Park Plaza that "I am owner, manager, and king of this hotel, and you'd better do what I say" (GRANDIOSITY).
HPI	He had checked into a four-star hotel a week ago with the intention of selling his screenplay to a Hollywood studio. Since checking in, he has **stayed awake for several nights** (DECREASED NEED FOR SLEEP) and has worked frantically on the script (INCREASED GOAL-DIRECTED ACTIVITY). He has charged several hundred dollars to his hotel room for caviar and full-course meals (RECKLESS SPENDING). Additionally, the bellboy reports that a different woman has spent the night in his room each day of the week (SEXUAL PROMISCUITY).
PE	Physical exam normal; neurologic exam normal; on mental status exam, **speech is rapid and pressured**; thought process is significant for **skipping from one idea to another in a loose and unrelated fashion** (FLIGHT OF IDEAS) and **going on frequent tangents without answering simple and directed questioning** (TANGENTIALITY); patient also reports that he is constantly thinking and can't keep up with his thoughts (RACING THOUGHTS).
Labs	Lytes/CBC: normal. TFTs: normal; RPR/VDRL nonreactive. UA: toxicology screen negative.
Pathogenesis	**No specific neurotransmitter systems have been definitively implicated** in bipolar I disorder. Concordance rates in monozygotic twins are higher than in most other psychiatric disorders, suggesting a **strong genetic component** to this illness.
Epidemiology	Prevalence is approximately 1%; males and females are equally affected. **Average age at onset is 25 years.**
Management	**Mood stabilizers** (lithium, valproic acid) and **neuroleptics** (olanzapine) constitute first-line pharmacotherapy. **Valproic acid** is often preferred for mania because it is associated with fewer side effects than lithium and because it can be "loaded" (i.e., large amounts can be given early in the course of treatment). For mania with agitation or psychosis, both **benzodiazepines** and traditional **neuroleptic drugs** can be used intermittently with mood stabilizers. **Antidepressants** can be used to treat future depressive symptoms, but caution should be exercised, as they may induce mania. Mood stabilizers are typically administered in conjunction with antidepressant therapy.

40 **BIPOLAR I DISORDER, MANIC TYPE**

Second- and third-line management includes the use of anticonvulsants such as carbamazepine, gabapentin, and lamotrigine. **Electroconvulsive therapy** is beneficial in refractory cases of mania or depression.

Complications

Approximately 90% of individuals who have a manic episode will have **future recurrences** without treatment. As the disease progresses, episodes are likely to occur with greater frequency and intensity, with less dependence on external stimuli for initiation. **Up to 10% to 15% of patients with bipolar disorder ultimately commit suicide.** Adverse effects of mood stabilizers vary; **lithium** is associated with weight gain, acne, hypothyroidism (monitor TFTs), nephropathy (monitor BUN/creatinine), fine tremor, diabetes insipidus, arrhythmias, and fetal cardiac defects. **Valproic acid** is associated with hair loss, weight gain, hepatotoxicity, pancreatitis, tremor, thrombocytopenia (rare), and fetal neural tube defects. **Carbamazepine** is associated with tremor, ataxia, hepatitis, aplastic anemia (1:20,000), Stevens-Johnson syndrome, and fetal neural tube defects.

Differential Diagnosis

■ **Bipolar I Disorder, Mixed Type** has episodes that meet the criteria for both depression and mania.

■ **Bipolar I Disorder, Depressed Type** is used to describe those patients with bipolar disorder whose most recent episode is depressive.

■ **Bipolar II Disorder** is characterized by hypomanic (less severe mania without psychosis) and full-blown depressive episodes. In bipolar II disorder, a history of depressive episodes must be present along with a history of at least one hypomanic episode.

■ **Major Depressive Disorder** lacks a history of manic episodes. The *sine qua non* of bipolar I disorder is the presence of at least one manic or mixed episode. A diagnosis of bipolar I disorder should be made in depressed patients if they have had one or more manic episodes at some time in the past.

■ **Substance-induced Mood Disorder/Acute Intoxication** due to substances such as cocaine, amphetamines, and PCP may cause agitation, pressured speech, and psychosis. Urine toxicology screen and substance abuse history are essential in diagnosis.

ID/CC A 33-year-old divorced woman returns to her primary care physician for follow-up after starting fluoxetine 4 weeks ago for a **depressed mood**.

HPI She had initially presented with 4 months of increasing **fatigue, difficulty concentrating, weight gain**, and **suicidal thoughts**. She now reports little change in her symptoms since starting her antidepressant. She spends most of the day sleeping in bed (HYPERSOMNIA) and finds that she does not enjoy her usual hobbies (ANHEDONIA).

PE VS: **bradycardia** (HR 56); hypotension (BP 80/40). PE: **skin coarse and dry; diminished reflexes throughout** (HYPOREFLEXIA); on mental status exam, **speech is slowed with deep voice**; patient can recall only one of three objects after 5 minutes (IMPAIRED SHORT-TERM MEMORY) and has difficulty counting backwards by sevens (IMPAIRED ATTENTION).

Labs **Elevated TSH** (20 μIU/mL); **low total T4** (2.2 μg/dL); elevated lipids.

Pathogenesis **Depression due to a general medical condition** is diagnosed if a medical disorder causes depression by a **known physiologic mechanism**. Common examples include **hypothyroidism**, cerebrovascular disease, multiple sclerosis, cancer (especially pancreatic and CNS), Cushing's disease, SLE, viral illness, Addison's disease, medications (beta-blockers, reserpine), sleep apnea, and Parkinson's disease. Clues to a possible medical etiology include no family history, older age of onset (after age 40), no recollection of previous depression, and a recent visit to another physician.

Epidemiology Up to 40% of patients with neurologic diseases such as Huntington's, Parkinson's, Alzheimer's, multiple sclerosis, and stroke experience severe depressive symptoms.

Management **Treatment of the underlying medical condition** should take priority; concurrent antidepressant therapy may be indicated if the depression is severe and slow to respond. In this case, treat hypothyroidism with thyroxine.

Complications Complications are related to the underlying medical illness. Psychiatric complications may include social and occupational

DEPRESSION DUE TO A MEDICAL CONDITION

disturbances, refusal of necessary medical procedures, and suicide.

Differential Diagnosis ■ **Major Depressive Disorder** cannot be diagnosed until an underlying medical condition is either ruled out or adequately treated.

ID/CC   A 70-year-old **woman** is seen by a consulting internist for **weight loss, fatigue**, and **insomnia** of **at least 2 weeks' duration**.

HPI   The patient says that she hasn't felt the same since she moved into a nursing home secondary to her failing health. She feels that since all her friends have passed away, she doesn't have anything to live for and **thinks about death frequently** (MORBID PREOCCUPATIONS). She denies any **suicidal plan** but feels that she'd be better off dead. She also reports **poor concentration** and **trouble remembering** things. She **no longer takes pleasure** in her old hobbies (ANHEDONIA) and often **feels worthless**. She also experiences intense **guilt** regarding past relationships.

PE   VS: normal. PE: mental status exam significant for **depressed mood, psychomotor retardation**, and **impaired short-term memory**.

Labs   Lytes/CBC: normal. TFTs: normal; RPR nonreactive.

Pathogenesis   Complex interactions of genetic, psychosocial, and neurobiologic factors are involved in major depressive disorder. Neurotransmitter systems that have been implicated include **serotonin** and **norepinephrine** (antidepressants are thought to exert their effect by affecting receptors or concentrations of either or both of these systems).

Epidemiology   **Females are affected more often** than males by a ratio of 2 to 1; lifetime prevalence risks range from 20% to 25% in women and from 7% to 12% in men.

Management   Psychotherapy and pharmacotherapy are equally efficacious for mild depressive syndromes. Pharmacologic therapy is most effective for more severe depression. **SSRIs have become first-line pharmacologic agents**. These include fluoxetine, sertraline, paroxetine, and citalopram. Common adverse effects include nausea, diarrhea, dizziness, restlessness, insomnia, anxiety, headache, decreased libido, and ejaculatory delay; adverse effects typically improve with time. Other first-line agents include **bupropion** (Wellbutrin), which primarily affects norepinephrine and dopamine neurotransmission; **venlafaxine** (Effexor) and mirtazapine (Remeron), which affect norepinephrine and serotonin neurotransmission; and nefazodone (Serzone), which affects serotonin neurotransmission. **Tricyclic antidepressants** are now considered by many as second-line agents owing to their

DEPRESSIVE EPISODE—MAJOR

adverse side effects and potential for fatal overdose; a baseline ECG is often recommended. Common agents include amitriptyline (Elavil), imipramine (Tofranil), desipramine (Norpramin), and nortriptyline (Pamelor). Side effects include sedation, postural hypotension, dry mouth, blurred vision, constipation, urinary hesitancy, quinidine-like effects on cardiac conduction, and decreased seizure threshold. Depression that fails to resolve with multiple 6-week trials at an adequate dosage of the above therapies can be treated with pharmacologic **augmentation strategies** (including lithium carbonate and thyroid hormone), **MAO inhibitors**, and **electroconvulsive therapy**.

Complications   Approximately 15% of depressed patients complete **suicide**.

Differential   ■ **Medical Conditions That May Cause Depression** include pan-
Diagnosis   creatic cancer, multiple sclerosis, stroke, and hypothyroidism. History, physical, and laboratory data are important to diagnosing underlying medical conditions.

■ **Dysthymia** involves symptoms of depression that have lasted at least 2 years and that do not meet the full criteria for major depressive disorder.

■ **Dementia** may be differentiated from cognitive impairments seen with depression (PSEUDODEMENTIA) on the basis of the temporal course of the illness and, ultimately, treatment response. Depression is generally characterized by more rapid onset and accompanied by marked affective distress (guilt, helplessness, depressed mood).

■ **Bipolar Disorder** requires a history of at least one manic or hypomanic episode.

■ **Adjustment Disorder with Depressed Mood** may be diagnosed when there is an identifiable psychosocial stressor and the symptoms do not meet the full criteria for major depressive disorder.

■ **Substance Use** may present with symptoms identical to those of major depression. Differentiating between a major depressive disorder and a **substance-induced mood disorder** is complicated, since they often coexist. In substance-induced mood disorders, the depressive symptoms are directly related to ingestion of substances.

■ **Bereavement** can be diagnosed when symptoms of a major depressive episode occur after the loss of a loved one. If the symptoms last more than 2 months and involve suicidal ideations, morbid preoccupations, or psychosis, then a diagnosis of major depression is made.

ID/CC   A 26-year-**old unmarried woman** presents to her primary care physician complaining of **feeling sad and hopeless**. She states that she has felt persistently depressed for **"at least** the last **2 years."**

HPI   The patient reports feeling **fatigued** at times and having poor self-esteem. However, she **denies any significant disturbance in sleep or appetite.** She **denies suicidal or homicidal ideation** and denies morbid ruminations. During the past 2 years of her illness, she has never been free of symptoms for more than 2 months at a time.

PE   Physical and neurologic exams normal.

Labs   Lytes/CBC: normal. TFTs: normal; RPR/VDRL nonreactive. UA: toxicology screen negative.

Pathogenesis   Although no clear etiology has been identified, psychological models and neurobiologic mechanisms have been implicated in dysthymic disorder.

Epidemiology   Prevalence is 4%; **females** are **affected more frequently** than males. Dysthymia is more common among unmarried persons and those with financial stressors. A major depressive episode may occur concurrently with dysthymic disorder, also known as **"double depression."**

Management   The treatment of dysthymia mirrors that of major depression. **Psychotherapy** (especially interpersonal and cognitive) and pharmacotherapy are clinically effective, but large controlled studies are lacking. Successful pharmacologic agents include **SSRIs** (fluoxetine, sertraline, paroxetine, fluvoxamine, citalopram), **tricyclic antidepressants** (imipramine, desipramine, amitriptyline), and **MAO inhibitors** (phenelzine, tranylcypromine).

Complications   Patients are at increased risk for **comorbid psychiatric illnesses. Substance dependence** disorders occur in approximately 15% of individuals with dysthymia. Other frequently observed comorbid conditions are **major depressive disorder** (so-called double depression) and **personality disorders.**

Differential Diagnosis

■ **Major Depressive Disorder** can be distinguished from dysthymia based on the number of criteria that are met for a major depressive episode and the duration of symptoms. In major depression, at least five of the nine criteria must be met (depressed mood, anhedonia, change in appetite, insomnia or hypersomnia, psychomotor agitation or retardation, fatigue or energy loss, feelings of worthlessness or excessive guilt, diminished concentration, and morbid preoccupations, including suicidal thoughts) over at least a 2-week period.

■ **Adjustment Disorder with Depressed Mood** involves symptoms that are due to an identifiable psychosocial stressor within the prior 3 months of the onset of symptoms. Also, the symptoms must resolve within 6 months after the removal of the identifiable stressor.

■ **Depression due to a Medical Illness** must involve a direct physiologic relationship between the illness and depression (e.g., Parkinson's disease, pancreatic cancer, hypothyroidism, CNS tumor, stroke).

ID/CC A 25-year-old **man** is brought to the emergency room following an automobile accident.

HPI The police report that the patient cut off another vehicle, leading to a major accident. The patient spent time in jail for vehicular assault. He demonstrates **a lack of remorse**, noting that "the idiot was driving too slowly and deserved what he got" (RECKLESS DISREGARD FOR THE SAFETY OF OTHERS). He also has a long history of **disorderly conduct** and **impulsive behavior**. He was **diagnosed with conduct disorder before the age of 15**, at which time he was regularly involved in physical altercations and other aggressive behaviors.

PE Minor abrasion to forehead and multiple tattoos; mental status exam within normal limits except for prominent sense of entitlement.

Labs UA: toxicology negative for cocaine, opioids, and PCP.

Imaging XR, cervical and thoracic spine: unremarkable. CT, head (noncontrast): negative.

Pathogenesis The etiology of antisocial personality disorder is multifactorial, likely involving an interaction between genetic predisposition and environmental stressors. **Risk factors** include **subnormal intelligence**, a history of **conduct disorder**, an **unstable home environment**, and **substance abuse**. A personality disorder is diagnosed only when the traits exhibited are stable over time. They must also be inflexible, maladaptive, and pervasive and must cause significant social or subjective distress.

Epidemiology Prevalence is 2%; **males** are **affected more than females** in a ratio of 3:1.

Management Antisocial personality disorder is sometimes amenable to self-help groups or to long-term psychotherapy with strict limit setting. Pharmacotherapy is reserved for comorbid illnesses. Antisocial personalities occasionally attempt to destroy and avoid therapeutic relationships. Inpatient groups are helpful in that patients cannot leave and peer interaction minimizes issues with authority.

Complications A significantly high proportion of people with antisocial personality disorder are found in the **prison** system.

Differential Diagnosis

■ **Narcissistic Personality Disorder** and antisocial personality disorder may both be characterized by a sense of entitlement and a desire for admiration; however, narcissistic personality disorder lacks the impulsivity, overt aggression, and disregard for the rights of others that characterize antisocial personality disorder.

■ **Conduct Disorder** is similar to antisocial personality disorder but is diagnosed if the patient is younger than 18 years or does not meet the long-term trait criteria of antisocial personality disorder.

■ **Substance Abuse** commonly coexists with antisocial personality disorder. However, antisocial personality disorder reflects a persistent maladaptive personality pattern that is present in the absence of any substance use. Toxicology screen and clinical history can help establish the temporal relationship of behavior and substance use.

ID/CC   A 38-year-old **woman** is brought to the ER after **cutting herself** on the left upper forearm.

HPI   She relates that she just had a fight with her boyfriend because he went to dinner with a female classmate. The patient has a long history of **self-mutilating behavior** after arguments or breakups with past boyfriends (FRANTIC EFFORTS TO AVOID REAL OR IMAGINED ABANDONMENT). Her **relationships have typically been stormy, intense, and unstable.** She has been hospitalized for overdoses and self-mutilation (RECURRENT SUICIDAL BEHAVIOR); cutting relieves her **chronic feelings of emptiness.** Later, while being seen by the chief resident, the patient becomes very angry and shortly thereafter is seen laughing pleasantly when her blood is drawn (AFFECTIVE INSTABILITY).

PE   Three superficial lacerations directly below left antecubital region; well-healed scars noted on both arms from past self-inflicted injuries.

Pathogenesis   No single etiology has been identified for borderline personality disorder (BPD); however, a biopsychosocial model involving the interaction between genetic and early childhood experiences has been implicated. Notably, patients with BPD often have a **history of physical and/or sexual abuse** during their formative years.

Epidemiology   Prevalence is 1% to 2%; **females** are **affected more than males.**

Management   Careful evaluation for comorbid axis I disorders (e.g., mood disorders, psychotic disorders, substance abuse disorder) should be undertaken during the initial assessment. **Dialectical behavioral therapy**, a modified version of cognitive behavioral therapy, is currently thought to be the most effective treatment for BPD. Pharmacotherapeutic approaches target symptoms of mood instability (treat with SSRIs), anxiety, impulsive behavior, and "mini-psychotic" episodes (treat with low-dose antipsychotics).

Complications   **Suicide** occurs in up to 10% of patients with BPD.

Differential Diagnosis   ■ **Mood Disorders (e.g., major depressive disorder, bipolar disorder)** often occur comorbidly with BPD, and distinguishing them may be difficult. BPD is characterized by a consistent maladaptive pattern of relationships and self-image beginning in adolescence, whereas mood disorders typically are not characterized by the stress-related paranoid ideations, dissociative experiences, or self-damaging impulsive behaviors found in BPD.

■ **Bipolar Disorder Type II**, which is characterized by depressive episodes and at least one hypomanic episode, can be distinguished by its intermittent nature, as opposed to the chronic, persistent symptoms of BPD.

■ **Histrionic Personality Disorder** may manifest with affective instability and need for attention; however, the self-destructive behaviors, dissociative experiences, and feelings of emptiness associated with BPD are lacking.

■ **Narcissistic Personality Disorder**, which is characterized by an elevated sense of importance and entitlement, can be distinguished from BPD by its impulsivity, lability of mood, and recurrent suicidality.

■ **Antisocial Personality Disorder** may manifest with a pattern of impulsivity and uncontrollable anger; however, the behaviors involve fighting, criminal acts, deceitfulness, and failure to conform to social norms.

ID/CC	A 42-year-old man is referred for a psychiatric evaluation by his employer to obtain a higher-level security clearance.
HPI	The patient works as a computer engineer for a nuclear submarine manufacturer that contracts with the government. He has **never had any close friends** and **rarely interacts with others** at work. He states that he is content with his work and has **little interest in social contacts.** When given the choice, the patient chooses **solitary activities** to keep busy. He has no prior history of mood disturbance, cognitive deficits, or psychotic symptoms.
PE	On mental status exam, **affect** is **flat and detached** and mood is euthymic; no evidence of delusions, hallucinations, or disorganized thought processes; attention, concentration, memory, and abstract thinking intact.
Pathogenesis	Genetic and psychosocial (i.e., detached parental figures, emotional withdrawal during childhood) models have been proposed for schizoid personality disorder (SZPD), but little evidence exists for either.
Epidemiology	Prevalence is estimated at 1% to 2%; more commonly seen in **males**.
Management	Patients with SZPD infrequently present to psychiatrists because of their aloof and detached nature. Furthermore, many individuals with SZPD are able to perform well at jobs that do not require significant social interaction, which keeps them from medical attention. **Group psychotherapy** has been a useful modality for some patients with SZPD.
Differential Diagnosis	■ **Avoidant Personality Disorder (AVPD)** can be distinguished from SZPD based on the patient's desire for social interactions. In AVPD, the patient seeks social intimacy but fears rejection and feelings of inadequacy, whereas in SZPD no interaction is desired.

■ **Schizotypal Personality Disorder** involves perceptual distortions (e.g., odd thinking, ideas of reference, illusions), eccentric appearance, and excessive social anxiety. |

SCHIZOID PERSONALITY DISORDER

ID/CC	A 26-year-old police officer is brought to the ER by his colleagues, who are concerned about a recent **change in his behavior**.
HPI	For 2 weeks he has been convinced that the other officers are trying to frame him. He thinks they want to kick him off the force because "they can read my dirty thoughts" (DELUSION). His wife confirms this history, adding that he has had a "short fuse" lately and has insisted that the blinds on the windows be kept closed. She also notes that he has been **suspicious** of his coworkers since having been passed up for a promotion **less than 1 month ago**.
PE	Neurologic and physical exams normal; on mental status exam, patient acts bizarre and answers questions in a loose and disorganized fashion (LOOSENING OF ASSOCIATIONS).
Labs	UA: toxicology screen negative.
Epidemiology	The disorder is uncommon. Fifty to eighty percent of patients diagnosed with brief psychotic disorder never have another psychotic episode.
Management	Administer **antipsychotics** (haloperidol, perphenazine, chlorpromazine, risperidone, olanzapine) to treat psychotic and agitated behavior. Short-acting **benzodiazepines** may also be used to treat anxiety and severe agitation. Supportive psychotherapy is a useful adjunct in the presence of precipitating stressors.
Complications	Brief psychotic disorder is associated with an increased risk of suicide. Acute administration of typical antipsychotic medications may be associated with extrapyramidal side effects such as dystonias, bradykinesia, and tremor. Coadministration of anticholinergic medications (e.g., benztropine) often prevents such adverse effects.
Differential Diagnosis	■ **Schizophreniform Disorder** is diagnosed when psychotic symptoms (hallucinations, delusions, disorganized behavior) are present for 1 to 6 months. ■ **Schizophrenia** should be diagnosed when psychosis persists for more than 6 months.

47 BRIEF PSYCHOTIC DISORDER

■ **Delusional Disorder** has symptoms that are present for at least 1 month, but the patient does not have prominent psychotic symptoms such as hallucinations, bizarre delusions, or grossly disorganized speech/behavior. Instead, the patient has a fixed and well-circumscribed delusion.

■ **Adjustment Disorder** does not have psychotic features.

■ **Mood Disorder with Psychotic Features** requires the presence of a mood disturbance (depression, mania) as well as symptoms that are mood congruent; that is, the patient experiences delusions and hallucinations with clearly depressive themes (e.g., delusions that the patient is rotting inside and that God hates him).

■ **Substance-induced Psychotic Disorder** can be diagnosed with a thorough history and toxicology screen.

ID/CC A 38-year-old man presents to a local police station complaining that the FBI has been following him unjustly (PERSECUTORY DELUSION) for **at least 1 month**.

HPI The patient believes that the FBI has placed him on surveillance since his visit to the White House earlier this year. Since then, he feels that the FBI has expanded its coverage of him, listening to his phone conversations and eavesdropping on his social interactions (NONBIZARRE DELUSIONS). He is successfully employed as a quality control manager for a chemical company, and his functioning has not been significantly impaired by the distractions. He is not particularly threatened by their actions but requests that the police intervene on his behalf.

PE Physical and neurologic exams normal.

Labs Normal.

Imaging CT, head: normal.

Pathogenesis The etiology of delusional disorder is unknown. The normal course of the disorder tends to be **chronic** and **unremitting**.

Epidemiology Delusional disorder is rare, and its prevalence has been estimated at 0.05%. The **persecutory type** of delusional disorder is the **most common** type.

Management Insight-oriented supportive psychotherapy may offer some benefit. Pharmacotherapy with pimozide may be helpful, although most delusions are refractory to treatment with neuroleptic agents. Always assess the patient's risk for endangering himself or others.

Differential Diagnosis ■ **Delusional Disorder, Erotomanic Type** is characterized by the false belief that another person is in love with the individual.

■ **Delusional Disorder, Grandiose Type** is characterized by delusions of exaggerated power, knowledge, wealth, or relationship to famous or religious figures.

■ **Delusional Disorder, Jealous Type** involves a false belief that an individual's partner is unfaithful.

DELUSIONAL DISORDER

■ **Delusional Disorder, Somatic Type** involves the delusion that the patient has a general medical condition.

■ **Delusional Disorder, Mixed Type** is used to describe a delusional disorder that involves more than one of the above types.

■ **Paranoid Personality Disorder** is characterized by pervasive distrust that extends into most relationships and is not encompassed by a single delusion.

■ **Chronic Paranoid Schizophrenia** and other psychotic disorders involve behavior and speech that are disorganized; negative symptoms, hallucinations, and bizarre delusions can also be used to distinguish between schizophrenia and delusional disorder.

■ **Major Depressive Disorder with Psychosis** involves mood-congruent delusions and major mood disturbances that occur concurrently.

■ **Dementia** involves delusions that are accompanied by multiple cognitive deficits.

■ **Delusion due to a Medical Condition or Substance Abuse** may be diagnosed with a thorough medical evaluation and toxicology screen.

ID/CC A **22-year-old** man is brought to the hospital by his parents secondary to increasingly **bizarre behavior** over the last **6 months**.

HPI The patient's parents relate a normal developmental history but note that he has always kept to himself and had **few friends** while growing up. Last year, during his junior year of college, his grades began to deteriorate and he took a semester off. Since then, his parents report that he **talks to himself, fails to maintain appropriate hygiene**, and shows no interest in going back to school. His parents add that he **no longer expresses emotions** (AFFECTIVE FLATTENING).

PE Physical exam normal; on mental status exam, patient reports hearing various voices speaking to him in a running conversation and frequently commenting on his actions (AUDITORY HALLUCINATIONS); he also reports receiving messages from God to combat the devil through the TV set (COMMAND HALLUCINATION); affect is flat, and thought process is difficult to follow.

Labs Lytes/CBC: normal. BUN and creatinine: normal; TFTs: normal; RPR nonreactive. UA: toxicology screen negative.

Imaging CT, head: slightly enlarged ventricles and mild cerebral atrophy.

Pathogenesis The **exact mechanism of schizophrenia is unknown**; genetic and neurodevelopmental factors likely play a central role. The **dopamine hypothesis** is based on **increased dopaminergic transmission in the mesolimbic area**; other neurotransmitter systems that have been implicated include GABA, glutamate, NMDA, and serotonin. The role of perinatal trauma and neurodevelopmental abnormalities is under research. Schizophrenia is categorized as paranoid, catatonic, disorganized, undifferentiated, and residual. In the **paranoid type**, the patient is preoccupied with paranoid delusions or frequent auditory hallucinations; other symptoms (e.g., disorganized behavior, affective blunting, catatonia) are not as prominent. This subtype is associated with the best prognosis. The **catatonic type** presents with bizarre posturing, a trancelike state with muscle rigidity (CATALEPSY), mutism, and repetition of words or phrases (ECHOLALIA). In the **disorganized type**, disorganized speech and behavior and inappropriate affect are prominent. The **undifferentiated type** is diagnosed when the symptom criteria for schizophrenia have been met (at least two of the following: hallucinations, delusions, disorganized behavior, disorganized speech, negative symptoms) but the patient does not fulfill the criteria for any other subtype.

SCHIZOPHRENIA

The **residual type** characterizes patients who previously met the criteria for schizophrenia but now demonstrate only attenuated symptoms of the disorder.

Epidemiology
Prevalence is 1%; males and females are affected equally. The average age of **onset is younger in males** (15 to 25) than in females (25 to 35). Risk factors include **family history**, birth complications (including viral infections), lower socioeconomic status ("downward social drift" is thought to be a consequence of severe social and functional deficits that lead people with schizophrenia to lives of relative poverty regardless of their pre-morbid socioeconomic status), and late winter or early spring births. Mortality due to suicide is approximately 10%, and more than **25% of schizophrenics will attempt suicide at some time in their lives**.

Management
There is controversy as to whether first-line pharmacologic management should consist of an **atypical** or a **typical neuroleptic**. Atypical neuroleptics (clozapine, risperidone, olanzapine, quetiapine, ziprasidone) have fewer extrapyramidal side effects, whereas the efficacy of typical neuroleptics (chlorpromazine, perphenazine, fluphenazine, haloperidol) has been better studied. Benzodiazepines (lorazepam, clonazepam, diazepam) can be useful for treating acute agitation and anxiety. Occupational and social skills training may prove useful as well, and education and therapy for the patient's family are helpful in decreasing hostile and negative affect, which may contribute to relapse. The gold standard for treatment-refractory schizophrenia is currently **clozapine**; however, its use is limited due to a **1% to 2% risk of agranulocytosis** and a consequent need for frequent blood monitoring. Use of olanzapine is also becoming more common because of its efficacy, lack of the traditional side effects of neuroleptics, and lack of risk for agranulocytosis. Electroconvulsive therapy is rarely used except in refractory or catatonic cases.

Complications
Untreated schizophrenia is devastating and can result in violent behavior and suicide. Serious adverse effects associated with neuroleptic treatment include restlessness (AKATHISIA), parkinsonism, acute dystonias, and neuroleptic malignant syndrome. The most detrimental long-term consequence of long-term traditional neuroleptic management is the development of involuntary motor movements (TARDIVE DYSKINESIA). Other adverse effects of neuroleptics include anticholinergic effects (blurred vision, dry mouth, urinary retention, constipation),

orthostatic hypotension, sedation, and hyperprolactinemia (gynecomastia, amenorrhea, sexual dysfunction). Newer atypical agents are associated with lower rates of extrapyramidal effects and tardive dyskinesia.

Differential Diagnosis

■ **Substance-induced Psychotic Disorders** must be distinguished from schizophrenia via a careful history to establish a temporal relationship of symptoms to drug use, coupled with urine toxicology and physical exam.

■ **Psychotic Disorder due to a General Medical Condition** must also be considered, as medical conditions such as CNS tumors or infections, temporal lobe epilepsy, SLE, HIV, and certain endocrine disorders may manifest with psychotic symptoms as well.

■ **Schizoaffective Disorder** is diagnosed when the criteria for both schizophrenia and an affective disorder (depression, mania, or mixed episode) are met. Additionally, there must be at least a 2-week period of psychotic symptoms in the absence of prominent mood disturbances.

■ **Schizophreniform Disorder** is diagnosed when the criteria for schizophrenia are present for > 1 month and < 6 months; it may progress to schizophrenia.

■ **Delusional Disorder** may be distinguished by the nature of the delusion (nonbizarre in delusional disorder) and the absence of auditory hallucinations and disorganized behavior.

■ **Brief Psychotic Disorder** involves psychotic symptoms that are present for longer than 1 day but for less than 1 month.

ID/CC	A 24-year-old man presents to a local plastic surgeon for corrective surgery of his "ugly nose."
HPI	He states he is frustrated and anxious with regard to his perceived defect. He stays at home and **avoids other people** (FUNCTIONAL IMPAIRMENT) because he fears they will stare at him. He also reports spending several hours a day **looking at his nose** in the mirror and often applies makeup to make his nose "less noticeable" (PREOCCUPATION WITH IMAGINED DEFECT). His past medical history is significant for **three rhinoplasties**.
PE	Nose appears symmetrical without gross abnormality.
Pathogenesis	The etiology of body dysmorphic disorder is unknown.
Epidemiology	Prevalence is uncertain. This disorder has been estimated to account for 2% of visits to plastic surgeons. Patients aged 15 to 20 years are most commonly affected, often with a positive family history for mood disorders and obsessive-compulsive disorder.
Management	**Psychotherapy** (cognitive, behavioral, and supportive therapy). **SSRIs** (fluoxetine, paroxetine, sertraline, fluvoxamine) may be the **most effective** pharmacologic treatment. It is unclear whether the efficacy seen with **tricyclic antidepressants** and **MAO inhibitors** is a result of treating an underlying depressive/anxiety disorder. **Antipsychotics** (haloperidol, perphenazine, olanzapine, risperidone) should be used when symptoms approach delusional intensity.
Differential Diagnosis	■ **Delusional Disorder, Somatic Type** is diagnosed when the belief is rigid, unshakable, and held with delusional intensity. Some cases may warrant a diagnosis of both body dysmorphic disorder and delusional disorder.
	■ **Anorexia Nervosa** should be considered when concern centers on body weight (weight < 85% of ideal body weight, fear of gaining weight, amenorrhea, restrictive or purging eating behaviors).

BODY DYSMORPHIC DISORDER

■ **Obsessive-Compulsive Disorder** is not diagnosed when the only symptom is preoccupation with appearance.

■ **Major Depressive and Anxiety Disorders** may coexist and exacerbate body dysmorphic disorder. Care should be taken to screen for the classic symptoms of depression and anxiety.

ID/CC	A 14-year-old **female** is brought to the ER **unable to move both lower extremities**.
HPI	The patient is accompanied by her mother, who reports that her daughter **witnessed a shooting** yesterday; her boyfriend was reportedly shot while standing next to her and then fell to her feet bleeding profusely (TEMPORAL RELATION TO STRESSFUL EVENT). The patient's mother says that the motor weakness came on several hours after the incident and has progressed to total paralysis below the waist. She is unable to walk but reports normal bladder function. Oddly, she seems **unconcerned with her symptoms** (LA BELLE INDIFFÉRENCE) and offers no explanation for them.
PE	Normal muscle tone in all extremities; 2+ reflexes globally; no flaccidity or fasciculations; sensory function intact throughout.
Labs	Normal.
Imaging	CT, lumbar spine: normal.
Pathogenesis	Psychological conflicts or stressors are typically associated with the symptoms in conversion disorder.
Epidemiology	More common in **females** and **lower socioeconomic groups**. Patients often present with sensory or motor complaints that are **unintentionally produced**, cannot be explained by an organic etiology, and are **usually associated with a psychological meaning**. For example, this patient may have been so afraid while witnessing the shooting that she wanted to run away. Because running away would also have meant abandoning her boyfriend (an impulse that is unacceptable to her), she unconsciously resolves this conflict by losing all strength in her legs, thereby preventing her from "running away."
Management	Allow patients to come out of their symptoms without invoking shame; **avoid telling patients that their symptoms are generated by mental processes**. Symptoms typically last from several days to a week and remit spontaneously. Occasionally, amobarbital ("TRUTH SERUM") or lorazepam (i.e., a benzodiazepine) is used to reduce anxiety and help engage the patient in therapy.

CONVERSION DISORDER

Differential Diagnosis

■ **Neurologic Illness (e.g., myasthenia gravis, multiple sclerosis, spinal cord trauma)** must be ruled out with appropriate medical approaches.

■ **Somatization** requires the presence of four pain symptoms, two gastrointestinal symptoms, one sexual symptom, and one pseudoneurologic symptom unrelated to a medical condition.

■ **Pain Disorder** involves only symptoms of pain with no apparent cause, or pain in excess of known organic pathology.

ID/CC	A 26-year-old health care worker presents to his primary care physician concerned that he has hepatitis. He reports that he drank water from a garden hose **approximately 6 months** ago and since then has experienced mild abdominal discomfort. The **preoccupation has persisted despite appropriate medical evaluation and reassurance**.
HPI	The patient denies any anorexia, diarrhea, or malaise. Additionally, he has no risk factors for hepatitis. Despite numerous benign medical workups and unremarkable lab values, he continues to fear that he has undetected hepatitis. He reports abdominal discomfort and gas after eating large meals, which he attributes to a flourishing hepatitis infection that is "destroying" his liver.
PE	Physical and neurologic examinations normal.
Labs	Lytes/CBC: normal. TFTs: normal; anti-HAV (IgG and IgM) negative; HBcAg negative; HBsAg negative; no heterophil antibodies.
Pathogenesis	Various psychological theories (e.g., low self-esteem, dependency needs, and displaced intrapsychic conflicts) and biologic theories (augmentation and amplification of bodily symptoms due to a lower threshold of discomfort, dysregulation of neurotransmitters) have been proposed.
Epidemiology	Prevalence in general medical clinics has been estimated to be as high as 5% to 10%; males and females are affected equally. Age at onset is usually between 20 and 30 years, and most patients have coexisting depressive or anxiety disorders.
Management	Careful assessment for comorbid psychiatric and medical illnesses. **Psychotherapy** (especially supportive, cognitive behavioral, psychoeducational) and pharmacologic therapy (i.e., **SSRIs**) have been used with limited success. Aggressive **treatment of underlying depressive and anxious symptoms** may decrease complaints related to hypochondriasis.
Differential Diagnosis	■ **General Medical Conditions** may present in a nonspecific manner; therefore, a thorough medical evaluation to rule out serious pathology is warranted in each case. ■ **Somatization Disorder** is characterized by multiple physical symptoms rather than by a predominant fear of having an

illness. Additionally, in hypochondriasis there is a misinterpretation of normal physical symptoms.

■ **Delusional Disorder, Somatic Type** can be distinguished from hypochondriasis based on the intensity of the conviction that one is ill; in delusional disorder, the individual is unable to consider the possibility that his or her ideas may be mistaken and that he or she is actually well.

■ **Other Major Psychiatric Disorders** it is important to distinguish affective and anxiety disorders with somatic preoccupations from hypochondriasis. Hypochondriasis should not be diagnosed if the patient's symptoms are better accounted for by a major psychiatric disorder.

ID/CC A **25-year-old woman** presents to an internist after leaving her previous primary care physician because he "hasn't helped even one of my medical problems over the last 2 years." She now has a new complaint of **abdominal bloating**.

HPI She has made **multiple visits** and phone calls to her primary care physician regarding her health over the past few years. She has also undergone extensive medical evaluations for symptoms, including **headaches, menstrual cramps, joint pains**, and substernal **chest pain** (PAIN SYMPTOMS). In addition, she has been evaluated for **nausea and diarrhea** (GASTROINTESTINAL SYMPTOMS). In the past year, she has seen specialists for **impaired sexual arousal** (SEXUAL SYMPTOM) and **double vision** (PSEUDONEUROLOGIC SYMPTOM), with unremarkable workups.

PE VS: normal. PE: mild abdominal tenderness; no peritoneal signs, masses, or distention; no other abnormalities noted.

Labs Lytes/CBC: normal. TFTs: normal; RPR/VDRL nonreactive; β-hCG negative for pregnancy; ESR: normal; rheumatoid factor and ANA negative.

Pathogenesis Factors implicated include genetic inheritance, abnormal regulation of the cytokine communication system within the nervous system, and abnormal neurophysiology.

Epidemiology Prevalence is 0.5%. The **age of onset must be before age 30** to meet criteria. Risks include poverty and low educational level; **females are affected more than males (5:1)**. Two-thirds of patients have coexisting mood, anxiety, or substance-related disorders.

Management Appropriate medical workup to **rule out valid medical pathology**. Routine brief office visits offer support and **reassurance**; additionally, the patient should have only one primary caretaker to help limit unnecessary workups. Reassurance that the patient's complaints, although valid, are not the result of a serious medical condition may help shift attention to the emotional components of the symptoms. Pharmacotherapy to target anxiety and depressive symptoms is often employed, although treatment of this disorder is in general very difficult. Psychotherapy significantly decreases hospitalization rates and expenditures.

Complications **Comorbid substance abuse** or other psychiatric disorders are seen in a large number of cases. Unnecessary surgical or medical procedures are often performed before this disorder is recognized.

Differential Diagnosis

■ **General Medical Conditions**: A thorough medical workup is indicated to rule out medical etiologies such as SLE, HIV, acute intermittent porphyria, irritable bowel syndrome, multiple sclerosis, myasthenia gravis, and endocrine disorders. It is important to note that multiple medical symptoms occurring late in life are often the result of a true medical illness.

■ **Undifferentiated Somatoform Disorder** applies to patients with one or more somatic complaints but fewer than the eight required for somatization disorder.

■ **Conversion Disorder** involves one or more symptoms of neurologic origin that are associated with psychological stressors.

■ **Hypochondriasis** is diagnosed when there is a preoccupation with fears that one has a serious medical illness. These preoccupations are based on a misinterpretation of physical symptoms.

■ **Factitious Disorder and Malingering** involve symptoms that are intentionally feigned for secondary gain (MALINGERING) or for assumption of sick role as a primary motivation (FACTITIOUS DISORDER).

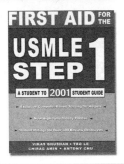
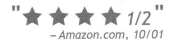
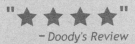
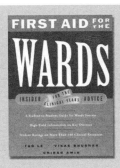
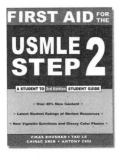
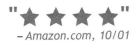
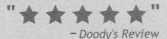
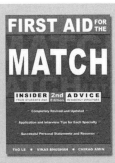